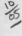

# The World's Best-Kept Beauty Secrets

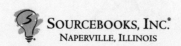

SOURCEBOOKS, INC.®
NAPERVILLE, ILLINOIS

# The World's Best-Kept Beauty Secrets

## What Really Works in Beauty, Diet, and Fashion

DIANE IRONS

Published by Sourcebooks, Inc.
P.O. Box 4410, Naperville, Illinois 60567-4410
(630) 961-3900
FAX: (630) 961-2168
www.sourcebooks.com

Originally published in 1997

Library of Congress Cataloging-in-Publication Data

Irons, Diane
The world's best kept beauty secrets: what really works in beauty, diet & fashion / Diane Irons
p. cm.
Includes bibliographical references and index.
ISBN 1-4022-0383-7
1. Beauty, Personal. I. Title.
RA778.I76 1997
646.7—dc21                                                                 97-1556

Printed and bound in Canada.
TR 10 9 8 7 6 5 4 3 2

# Also by Diane Irons

The World's Best-Kept Diet Secrets

Age-Defying Beauty Secrets

Diane Irons' 14-Day Beauty Boot Camp

911 Beauty Secrets

Bargain Beauty Secrets

Teen Beauty Secrets

# Dedication

## To my mother and father

for their love, guidance, and work ethic.

# Table of Contents

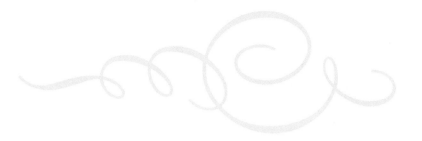

# Acknowledgments

I need to thank my family, friends, and colleagues who have supported my dedication to my work and have been patient when I must "drop out" to conduct research and create my message.

The lovely "guinea pigs" who are always willing to try yet another recipe, product, or idea—this patience and enthusiasm especially extends to my mom, sisters Stephanie and Leah, Kirk's Elizabeth, sister-in-law Ginny, and her daughter Kim. I always appreciate your feedback and honesty.

My admiration and gratitude goes out to the many women who have come to me for help and allowed me the pleasure of working with them. Placing yourself in my hands is both humbling and the joy of my work.

I appreciate the dedication and professionalism of my publisher, Sourcebooks, their flexibility and understanding. Bethany Brown, you have great vision and creativity.

Finally, to all those women I have yet to meet—but who have touched me with their stories and honesty—you are always in my thoughts, and help me to keep trying to find a better way to reach you.

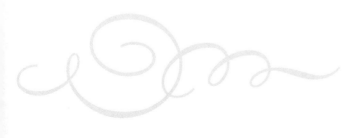

# Introduction

When I was first inspired to write *The World's Best-Kept Beauty Secrets*, it was because I had gathered years of interviews, tips, and important information as a model, trainer, and fashion and beauty journalist. Although I had the opportunity to share this information in my TV and radio work as well as in ongoing speaking engagements, I wanted to document this information in a permanent location accessible to anyone and everyone who aspired to look and feel better about themselves without spending a lot of time or money.

I thought at the time that I had found out everything there was to live a beautifully well-rounded—yet affordable—existence, but instead, found that as I headed on book tour to share these secrets, the enthusiasm of what I had found inspired others to share their own "best-kept beauty secrets." Some came from the makeup artists and professional stylists who worked with me on tour, while many others were from readers, fellow guests sitting in the green room with me, and tips from interested experts on new ground-breaking research.

Then as I continued my research and consulting, I found that I was adding to my repertoire of tips and secrets on what seemed like a daily basis. I continued to interview women who shared their beauty routines with me and just had to document them. Some were tried and true for generations, while others were the result of a lot of: try this; no, that doesn't work; okay, I'll live with that scar for a while; so what about this? Let's see what happens when I mix these products together. Voila!

Then there's the constantly changing market out there. New resources pop up while others just fade away or are no longer relevant.

Fashion and style can also make their mark and then leave the scene. Sometimes they just go away for a little while, and then there's those "What we were thinking?" trends.

Rules change, and what worked yesterday may need some rethinking to apply today. Other things may just need to be restructured a bit.

Whatever the reason, I found myself making these changes as I went along, adding to the bargains, finding new supplements and stories, and literally sticking them all over the chapters or calling my editor to see if I could stick something in for the next printing. Rather than attempt to give out this information during my speaking engagements, I have decided to totally update *The World's Best-Kept Beauty Secrets* so that although it remains basic and classic in its

approach, it can now be considered totally accurate with its resources and data, as well as its impetus for creative thinking.

I've also given you an entire section of my prized collection of beauty recipes that you will find relaxing and enjoyable. Although many of these recipes are very close to those prized and pricey treatments from the world's most renowned spas and salons, I have chosen the ones that will be most practical and effective for you. I want you to be able to perform these remedies in the privacy of your own home, with easy-to-find ingredients that won't allow you any guilt for time or money spent.

I hope that this new and updated information will be just what you need to access your own unique and spectacular beauty and style.

*chapter*
# one

# Attitude

# You Are What You Project!

Welcome to the best-kept secrets of the world's most alluring women. The models, actresses, and celebrities I have been privileged to work with have one trait that causes them to stand out in a crowd—the attitude they project to the world. These women that you see on the street, on the movie screen, or adorning the pages of your favorite magazines are not the most beautiful women ever created. But don't tell them that!

All women can be truly beautiful. The sad fact of life is that there are some potentially lovely women out there who are holding on to some very old myths. I have worked with "displaced housewives" who decided to throw all their beauty, health, and diet routines away because the routines were too self-indulgent or complicated. So what do they do with their extra time? They spend it adorning their homes or families. Hello? What about your inner house? It is not necessary to give up yourself to love someone else; it is only when you truly love and respect yourself that you can give to others freely.

## Make the Time

Create precious time for yourself by setting the alarm clock thirty minutes earlier than usual. Begin rituals for yourself that will become as important to you as breathing. If you really don't think that you have enough time during the day, then take it from the minutes wasted on phone calls, shopping, or mindless TV surfing.

## Keep It Simple

Begin a "housecleaning" on your body, closet, handbag, cosmetics, and anything else that keeps you from feeling good about yourself and your life.

## Stand Up Straight

This sounds so ridiculously simple, but it's one of the most evidential traits of those women we so admire. Stand against a wall with head, shoulder blades, and heels touching, and buttocks pushed into the wall. Walk away without changing this position. A great posture is a wonderful beginning for your attitude adjustment.

While you're at it, why don't you adjust those droopy bra straps? This will help "pick up" both those drooping shoulders and those downward-spiraling breasts.

## Be the Star of Your Own Show

*You* should be what people notice. Your cosmetics and clothes should not compete for attention with each other, or with you. Stay with the basics, but invent your own style. If you like the color red, then use it as a consistent accent piece in your wardrobe. Do you have a special collection of pins or bracelets? Show them off; make them your signature. But definitely do not attempt to wear more than two pieces at a time.

## Make an Effort

You owe it to your self-esteem, your family, and your friends to try! After all, you don't like to look at a messy house or office all day, do you? Don't you really love and admire majestic artwork? A lovely flower arrangement? Become your own canvas, and recreate yourself.

## Have It Your Way

After years of telling us what to wear and how to wear it, designers have finally accepted that women are not going to be dictated to any more. Finally, after huge rebellions (along with lagging retail sales) in department stores across the country, there is a choice in hemlines, fabrics, and so much more. The result? If you have great legs, feel free to show them off! If you have a lovely waist, accentuate it with a long and elegant ensemble. Play up your good features, and hide away those "less-than-perfect" areas.

## Learn to Trust Your Mirror

Most of us believe only what others tell us, not what we see in the mirror. That's why we desperately seek compliments and depend on other people's feedback. Real "beauties" rely on their mirror and accept everything they see. When they behold great hair, they enjoy their "good hair day." You won't find these women concentrating on the two pounds they gained from last night's dessert.

## Don't Be So Modest

While we are encouraged to go out and look our best, we're not supposed to admit that we're trying. Going that "extra yard" for beauty is sometimes perceived as prideful vanity. In addition, some women worry that they may attract the wrong attention, but wallflowers belong only on walls!

# Don't Act or Dress Your Age

Every beautiful woman that I have interviewed seemed to possess the same trait: agelessness. If I hadn't been privy to their backgrounds, I would have been hard-pressed to put a "number" on them. You know who these women are—you've seen them in a magazine or on TV. You know they are about your age, but they look so much "better." Don't necessarily jump to the conclusion that they've had extensive plastic surgery. That is not always the case.

How do you begin your own "timeless" appearance? Pick up a magazine that might be geared to a different age demographic. Shop at a different store or department than you usually do. Find a mentor, someone whose style you've always admired, to help you develop your new look.

*Almost everything we do is based on appearance. The pursuit of beauty is as old as time. Cute babies are held longer. We love flowers for their "beauty."*

# Start a Journal

The first step to finding your way back to you is to start a daily journal. Keep your daily activities and thoughts as a reliable thermometer to your current state of thinking. Use it to keep track of what you're eating, wearing, and feeling.

# Find Your Energy Level

Every person possesses an inner clock. Don't rely on the time of day to tell you when to eat, when to rest, etc. Let your body do the talking! It never fails to give you signs that tell you what it needs.

Know when to let go! You're not in charge of the universe.

# Set Goals

Don't get overwhelmed in the steps to your transformation. Set standards and goals in baby steps. This is especially important if you've somehow lost yourself along the way. It could be as small as "I will lose five pounds by the end of the month" or "I will devote one hour a day just for me." Sit back, close your eyes, and visualize yourself as slimmer, happier, or more assertive.

Beauty begins with self-acceptance.

Look in the mirror, smile, and say "hi!"

## No-Brainer

Have one or two outfits that you know make you look terrific and require no thought. Keep no more than five cosmetics that can take you out the door and don't have to be color coordinated. Keep one overcoat that will look stylish, take you out the door with dignity, and hide anything!

## Keep Moving!

Don't stay frozen in time. It is such an easy and comfortable place to get stuck. Keep a look that is absolutely your style, but keep reinventing that look to keep up with the times. You know who the guilty ones are. You've seen that woman who wears that seventies Farrah Fawcett hairdo, when not even Farrah herself has kept that same look. Or better yet, that friend who was mod in the sixties and refuses to believe that the revolution is over!

# Learn to Forgive

Get back to self-acceptance. Did you break your diet? That just means that you are human. Why is it that it's so much easier to forgive others and not ourselves? Let it go! When you overspend a bit, maybe that's just what you needed at that time to build your spirits. If you find it difficult to forgive others, remember that even the most well-intentioned person can hurt your feelings. Don't dwell on it. Don't let it stay with you, or it will convert itself into a binge, spending spree, or something far more depressing. Throw it away, and get on with your life *today*!

# Meditation Is a Beauty Ritual

I have had the privilege of working with some big names in the modeling and celebrity world. Each of these great stars possessed the unique ability to go into some kind of trance when sitting behind that mirror. This is a concept that I have found to be a perfectly relaxing and enjoyable way to start the day.

# *I Double Dare You*

Remember that game we used to play as children? Whether it's just getting a manicure or changing your hair color, just a little something new or different can create a brand-new mind-set. Oh yes, of course, you can always change it back if you don't like it. But you may love the new you and wonder why you didn't try it sooner!

# Self-Portrait

Drawings are our subconscious speaking to us.
Take a pencil or crayon, and draw a picture of yourself.

Ask yourself what your drawing says about you.

1. Did you take up the whole page?

2. Are you in the corner?

3. Are any of your body parts missing?

4. Are you wearing clothes?

5. What kinds of clothes are you wearing?

6. Are you wearing shoes?

7. Are any of your body parts out of proportion?

8. What would you name your drawing?

Whenever I speak to groups or work with clients, I often use this self-test. It reveals what we need to know in order to change our image and esteem issues.

The most evidential self-portrait results were the ones done by teenagers and homemakers reentering the workplace. They were most likely to draw themselves without body parts, grotesque bodies, or as being practically invisible, taking up only a small corner of the page.

# Skin

# Water

Water is the number one beauty treatment favored by women of every age. You cannot create beauty without beginning with a clean, clear palette.

Forget the very expensive imported waters. If you don't drink at least eight to ten glasses a day, you are depriving yourself of the best beauty treatment on earth.

Japanese women spend twice as much time and money on their skin than any other women in the world.

# The Sun Is Your Skin's Number One Enemy

You should always make sun protection a priority. Use a sunscreen formulated for your skin along with your moisturizer. Much of the evidence of aging—rough skin, wrinkles, age spots, etc.—are really the result of too much sun. Always apply lots of it not only to your face, but slather it on the neck, hands, and hairline.

# Cleansing

The first rule of beautiful skin is to stop overcleansing it. This is an unnecessary habit, especially true of women in this country. Unless you've been up all night digging ditches (you poor dear!), your face is not dirty. Your morning routine should be nothing more than reactivating last night's moisturizer with a splash of warm water or milk. Why milk? Milk is a lactic acid and will allow your face to receive a natural acid treatment.

Please be aware that many of the acids on the market today are synthetic acids that have caused problems with some women. There have been reports of everything from sensitivity rashes to permanent scarring. Be careful of the chemical acids you use, and when you can, substitute nature's acids in your cleansing routine. In addition to milk, consider these natural acids:

1. Pineapple juice

2. Lemon juice

3. Tomatoes

4. Most citrus fruits

# *Toning*

Toning is your second step, and an important one. The purpose of using a toner is to remove residue soap, moisturizer, and oil. You can spend a lot for a toner (up to $20 and more at some cosmetic counters), or you can do what many famous models do. Carry around lemons. They are refreshing and more effective than those silly toners that contain only a little lemon but lots of chemicals.

Other inexpensive alternatives:
1. Rose water

2. Witch hazel

3. Hydrogen peroxide

4. Or try the following refreshing tea tonic: Mix 2 teaspoons of green or chamomile tea with 1/2 cup water. Saturate a cotton ball, and apply all over the face. Allow it to remain on the skin until it evaporates.

NOTE:

There's never any reason to rinse this or any toner off.

# Moisturizing

I am happy to pass on one of the most important ways to save money. It is not necessary to spend a lot on a moisturizer. Good basic moisturizers can be found in any drugstore. Just learn to read the labels, and look for these low-cost ingredients.

### Lipids
Listed as ceramides, cerebrosides, or sphingo lipids.

### Essential fatty acids
Listed as sunflower oil, grapeseed oil, and primrose oil.

### Sunscreen
Now available in many moisturizers as a step-saver.

## tip

Don't buy a vitamin E, A, or C enhanced moisturizer. Go to your local pharmacy, and purchase these vitamins in capsule form. Get as much potency as is available. Prick open the capsule, and add it to your moisturizer. You'll get all the benefits of the expensive cosmetic creams without the extra chemicals or expense.

# Add Water

You'll find most moisturizers more effective when applied to damp skin. It forms a thin film that will trap moisture in the skin. Evening is the most important time to take care of your skin. The sleeping hours are when your face is away from makeup, dirt, pollution, etc., and is free to rejuvenate. Your evening regime is also effective and useful in de-stressing your entire psyche to prepare you for the best treatment of all: beauty sleep.

Just follow these steps:

## 1. Cleanse

Make it easy on yourself, your skin, and your purse by using just one product to remove both makeup and dirt. If your skin is dry, use a lotion or cream-based product that leaves behind emollients (it will feel like a light film on your face). If your skin is "normal to oily," use a gel cleanser or a very mild facial soap. Even though your skin may be very oily, be sure to use a gentle soap like Neutrogena or Dove. Never use a deodorant soap on your face or neck. If your skin is particularly sensitive, don't even use it on your body!

## 2. Exfoliate

I cannot overstate the need for this step. What is exfoliating? It is very much like peeling an onion or removing tiles off a roof. Exfoliating is necessary to get blood flowing into the face, as well as to remove grime.

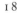

## HERE'S WHAT TO USE

- Take a packet of sugar (raw sugar works the best), add a couple of drops of olive oil to make it easier to spread, and gently rub it into the creases of your face.

- Open a packet of instant oatmeal and mix it with water to create a paste. Rub this mixture into your face, and rinse off the residue. I would suggest that you use instant oatmeal on your face, and the traditional old-fashioned oatmeal to exfoliate the entire body.

- Rub sea salt (available in health food stores) all over both your body and face. You'll love its invigorating effects.

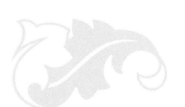

## 3. Masks

My favorite face mask is the result of my most memorable investigative reporting story. I had been informed that those very expensive spas that charge hundreds of dollars for "herbal wraps" were using mud. Now the inside "scoop" is that these "chichi" places were not using some exotic mud from the Dead Sea, but a formula created from kitty litter.

Okay, we've all heard of clay masks. Clay is perfect for detoxifying the skin. What I discovered is that these so-called "mud" or "clay" treatments used by some salons is nothing more than kitty litter. The catch is that the bag must be marked "100 Percent Natural Clay." It cannot contain any chemicals, additives, or clumping materials. The good news is that this type of kitty litter is generally the least expensive on the market.

## HOW TO USE IT

Take about a tablespoon of the dried clay and reconstitute it with a small amount of water. Mud is mud is mud! I don't care if it comes from the great Springs of Italy (and if it does, you'll spend about $60 a jar) or from your local grocery store. At less than $2 a bag, detoxify your entire body with it. I have worked with the most fabulous celebrities who swear by my kitty litter facial, including top makeup artists. Although they love this facial, they know that their clients may be a little reticent to try such an unorthodox facial. So they pour the kitty litter into an attractive container. You might want to do the same at your house to avoid strange looks. Potpourri jars make delightful hideouts for your new find.

I have demonstrated this several times on national TV shows with people from the audience, and not one person has ever told me that it felt anything but absolutely refreshing. It actually possesses a kind of pleasant, minty feel. Minerals in the mud also benefit the skin.

Please don't try to dig up the mud from your yard. Real mud is dirty and contains organisms that harbor diseases.

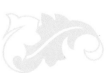

# Other Face Masks to Try

## Ultimate Cleansing Mask

In a blender or food processor, grind 1 cup of oatmeal to a powder. Add 3 drops of almond oil, 1/2 cup of milk, and 1 egg white. Continue to blend together, and apply. Rinse off after 20 minutes.

## Peach and Brandy

Mash up a peach (use ripe, canned, or frozen) and mix in a tablespoon of brandy. Leave it on for 20 minutes, and rinse off.

## Tomato Mask

For oily skin, mash up a ripe tomato and leave it on for 15 to 20 minutes. Rinse with warm (not hot) water.

## Banana Mask

Mash up a very ripe banana. Add just enough honey to make a soft pulp. Apply over face and hair. This is such a great firming mask that aging movie stars have been known to put it in the cups of their bras to make their breasts "perky."

Just make sure that you don't add too much honey, and that you use a sturdy bra. I recently did a TV show where I attempted to use a lacy bra. Needless to say, it was a little messy!

## Honey Mask

Apply pure honey (straight from the bottle) to your face and neck. Allow it to set until dry (about 15 minutes). Rinse with very warm water.

## Milk of Magnesia Oil-Absorbing Mask

Apply it straight from the bottle. Let it dry for about five to ten minutes. Rinse off with warm water.

Gently pat face dry with fluffy towel.

## Pepto-Bismol

This is a face mask particularly suited for those with sensitive skin. In the same way that this product coats the stomach, it gently caresses the face.

Apply it straight from the bottle with a cotton swab. Allow it to dry and rinse with cool water. It's as refreshing as a cool summer breeze.

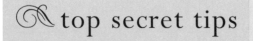 top secret tips

## To Revitalize and Nourish the Skin

Soak whole dried beans or lentils (fresh are best) overnight. Mash and add a small amount of honey. Apply over face and neck. Leave it on for about 5 minutes and rinse with tepid water.

## Tone Up Tired Skin

Make up a smooth pulp of crushed cucumbers, and gently pat all over face and neck. Pull up your hair and apply a little bit behind the ears and behind the neck. This facial is absolutely fabulous for oily skin and clogged pores.

Mix 1/4 cup vodka with the juice of one fresh lemon. Dab it on the face, neck, and chest area with a cotton swab. It's not necessary to rinse off. Let the air evaporate it. The less rubbing that you do to the face the better.

# More Beauty Tricks from the Kitchen Cupboard

## Clove Oil Cleanser

Combine equal amounts of clove oil (a natural astringent), chamomile (to maintain skin pigment), and eucalyptus (decongests the skin). Massage gently into the skin by making a circular motion with the tips of your fingers, and rinse.

## Crisco

Right from the can, Crisco is a big secret among beautiful women. Use it to remove makeup and as a highly effective moisturizer. Hospitals even use it to treat psoriasis and eczema. They are known to disguise it as cream "C."

## Wheat Germ Oil

Available in health food stores and some supermarkets, wheat germ oil is effective in keeping the skin elastic and preventing and treating stretch marks. Pregnant women should definitely use it in the tummy and breast areas.

## Sweet Almond Oil

Available in supermarkets, almond oil is ideal for removing makeup, helping eyelashes grow, and as a moisturizer for extremely dry skin. It also soothes sunburned skin.

# Bathing

Add some baking soda to your bath (about half a box). It will soothe itching skin, irritation, and sunburn.

Use Epsom salts (about one-half pound) to relax muscles and relieve swelling.

Try some instant oatmeal (or grind any other to a powder) in the tub to get rid of sunburn.

Apple cider vinegar in the bath will invigorate the body and fight fatigue.

Adding a spoonful of honey is said to help insomnia.

Combine a cup of instant milk powder with 3 drops of almond oil. Soak for at least 15 minutes, then using a coarse wash cloth or loofah, rub vigorously to exfoliate (remove) dead skin. Your skin will absolutely glow and shine!

Should you start to feel a cold coming on, take a teaspoon of mustard powder and add it to a hot bath. You just might fight off the cold.

Orange slices in the bath are uplifting and beat any aromatherapy available today.

Through the ages red wine has been used as a beauty treatment. Since it is a tannic acid, many beauties use it as an acid-based toner.

# Sharing Beauty Treatments with Our Animal Friends

For years models have been sneaking into feed supply stores and equestrian shops for Bag Balm and Hoof Maker. Now these beneficial products are being sold in drugstores and mass merchandisers everywhere.

Hoof Maker is as it sounds, a hoof conditioner for horses. However, it softens cuticles, heels, and other rough spots. Horse trainers came upon this terrific product by seeing their own positive results. It seems that their nails and cuticles were stronger, longer, and more resilient.

Bag Balm is an emollient used to soothe those poor cow's udders that take such a licking in those milking machines. This stuff (it's very inexpensive) is wonderful on chapped lips and as extra protection during cold weather on hands and face. It's a must for skiers.

Kalaya Oil is one of the oddest moisturizers ever to hit the cosmetic market. It is derived from the "fat back" of the rare Australian bird, the emu. This moisturizer lessens the signs of aging by trapping moisture in the skin.

# Moisturizer Know-How

1. Don't over-moisturize. Use cream on specific areas. You may not need it all over your face. The cheeks and forehead tend to be drier than the chin.

2. Choose the right formula for your skin type. More than half of all women misdiagnose their skin type, believing it to be very oily or very dry. It's highly unusual for a woman's skin to be either. If moisturizer is too heavy, the result is clogged pores. Moisturizing techniques need to be changed as the seasons change.

3. Get more from your moisturizer by circulating the skin. Gently tap the face by pretending your face is a piano, and you're "playing" it.

4. Any moisturizer can be stretched by first applying a film of natural vegetable oil as a base.

5. Wait until a moisturizer is completely absorbed before applying foundation. However, if a foundation is a bit dry, moisturizer can loosen it up a bit. The foundation will go on more smoothly.

# Cellulite

We now know that diet works and thigh creams don't when it comes to cellulite. So what else can we do besides just staring at it? Here are some simple steps:

1. Eat lots of fresh fruit and vegetables (preferably raw).
2. Keep away from processed foods.
3. Drink lots of water to rid cells of toxins.
4. Stay away from carbonated beverages (even low-calorie).
5. Avoid alcohol, which negatively affects the liver, the body's main detoxifier and filter.
6. Try to walk or jog at least three times a week for 30 to 45 minutes.
7. Scrub the skin with a bristle brush or loofah. Brush in slow sweeps, always toward the heart. There are gloves and mitts available to do this, but they're not necessary. Try to do this at least five minutes a day.

Models are using their morning coffee grounds to massage their cellulite areas. The main ingredient in expensive cellulite creams is caffeine, so it makes a lot of sense. Simply sit on the edge of your bathtub, and rub the coffee grounds into those pesky areas. It could get messy, so make sure that you have a few newspapers laid out under you!

8. Copy the expensive herbal wraps offered by top spas. Mix 1 cup of corn oil with 1/2 cup of grapefruit juice and 2 teaspoons dried thyme. Massage into hip, thigh, and buttock areas. Cover with plastic wrap to lock in body heat. For extra results, lay a heating pad over each area for about five minutes.

# Stages of Cellulite

Do you have it? How bad is it? Cellulite does have a way of progressing like a bad fungus.

## Test

Cellulite can be diagnosed by using the skin pinch-and-roll technique. Gently take a large fold of normal skin and rub it between your thumb and forefinger. The skin should appear smooth.

Now repeat this test on areas where you think you have cellulite. You may have cellulite in the following stages:

## Stage 1

The skin will show no visible signs, but bruises and cuts may be slow to heal in this area.

## Stage 2

Looking closely at the skin, you'll see broken veins and skin discoloration. Bruises will appear after a small hit. When pinched, the skin will feel thicker and slightly tender with slight ripples.

## Stage 3

Even without pinching the skin, you'll see evidence of an orange-peel appearance.

## Stage 4

The skin will appear puckered, and is cold to the touch. Broken veins will be present, and bruising can occur spontaneously.

## Stage 5

Not only will you feel cold areas, but hot areas will also be evident.

## Stage 6

Large lumps of fat are honeycombed in fibers, distorting the appearance of the cellulite area.

# Quick Skin Pick-Me-Up

Do you need a quick glow to your skin and an all-over healthier look? Bend over at the waist, as far as you can possibly go, and hold to the count of thirty. Scientists have proven that this very simple stance boosts circulation to both face and scalp, speeding up the turnover of skin cells and reducing the possibility of breakouts. Benefits vary depending on the time of day you choose.

## Morning

It helps you to focus on a busy day and awakens the mind and body.

## Noon

This is the time for a midday boost.

## Night

It helps you unwind, and gets your heart rate and your breathing back to where they should be.

Try to get your head in the proximity of your knees. It's okay to bend your knees until you get used to the position. Steady the stance by clasping your hands behind your back. Still can't seem to do it? Just lie over the side of your bed (head down).

**tip** Retin-A is doing for stretch marks what is has done for the face. Researchers have found that women using this prescription drug on stretch marks reduced them by 14 percent after six months of continued use.

# Blemished Skin Aids

Tincture of Benzoin
Oatmeal
Yogurt
Strawberries
Tea tree oil

# Fade Cream

Make your own concoction to lighten age spots and sun-damaged upper chest. Mix the juice of 1 lemon, 1 lime, 2 tablespoons of honey, and 2 ounces of plain yogurt. Gently massage into each spot. Use at least once a week.

# To Squeeze or Not to Squeeze

If you decide to squeeze a pimple, be very gentle, pressing until it bleeds may rupture tissue and cause scarring. Make sure that skin is clean and warm, wrap your fingers in tissue, and apply light pressure. Dab over it with tea tree oil.

# Face-Lift

There are ways to lift your face, both on a cumulative and temporary basis. For years models, actors, and actresses have been relying on the shark's liver oil and yeast contained in some hemorrhoidal creams. These are the same ingredients that can be found in expensive "firming" creams sold at expensive cosmetic counters. Just what these creams do for those other areas (takes down the swelling and shrinks tissues) is what they do for under-eye bags, droopy jowls, etc. Makeup artists won't do a makeover without it. Rock stars, Hollywood's big names, and other celebrities won't go on the road without a supply of it. Many of the people you believe have had plastic surgery have been using it for years.

If you object to the medicinal smell, simply mix it with a small amount of your regular moisturizer. If you do need to use it and head out the door right away, just dab a little perfume in front of each ear to diffuse any odor. I once interviewed a very handsome actor in his mid-fifties, and could not get over how great he looked. However, I was aware of a certain aroma that I recognized wafting from his direction. If you find that this product works for you, I suggest that you use it at night in the privacy of your own bedroom.

If you are heading out to a special event and want to tighten your face a bit, use this quick fix:

Beat 1 egg white to a froth. Apply all over face, paying special attention to the eye area, chin, and jaw. Allow it to dry (it should take no longer than ten minutes) and ever so lightly rinse it off. Don't waste your money on temporary lifting creams. The egg white lift is just as effective as any "face-lift in a bottle" I have ever tried.

## Eyes

Thin cucumber slices used as compresses over closed eyes will relieve sore, puffy eyes.

Raw potato slices contain potassium to take away dark circles under the eye.

Inexpensive tea bags (make sure that they're cool to the touch) on the eyes make good eye refreshers because of the tannic acid. Don't use herbal tea bags, because most don't contain tannic acid. Try such brands as Red Rose and Lipton, or even better, generic brands.

# Neck

The neck is often one of the most neglected areas, yet it's the first place where the signs of aging appear. A certain amount of wrinkling and sagging is inevitable, but there is a lot you can do to not only improve the appearance of your neck now, but minimize future problems.

Always take your cleanser and creams over the entire throat area, rinsing thoroughly. Make certain to apply all creams with firm upward strokes.

# Knees and Elbows

The skin on knees, elbows, and heels can easily look discolored and dead. Here's a bleaching mask that really works wonders. Don't you even think of wearing a short skirt without first applying this mixture.

Add the juice of 3 lemons to 1 cup of powdered milk. Use just enough water to make a thick paste. Leave the mixture on for 20 minutes. Scrub off briskly with a loofah or sponge.

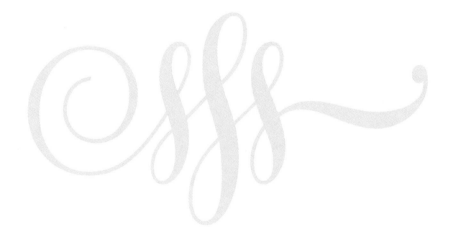

# chapter three

# *Hair*

# A Good Hair Day

So what do you want from your hair? You probably want it to behave. You want it to have volume. You want it to shine. That's just how you decide what you need in a hair product. The number one question I'm asked when it comes to hair:

"Is there a difference between expensive hair salon products and drugstore items?"

After all these years of research, I still find that there are no immediate answers. I have tried them all (and have the split ends to prove it), yet have not come up with anything that beats the natural-based formulas.

Because everyone's hair is unique, it is necessary to experiment a bit. The key is to purchase the smallest size available (travel sizes are ideal), and see what works. We've all seen the big sales and ripped out the coupons. What good is a big vat of that product going to be if it makes your hair look like a miniature haystack?

Here's all you'll need for beautiful hair. And I pray that you never again overspend, buy a useless product, or have a "bad hair day."

## Find a Stylist You Like and Trust

Ask a friend or even a stranger on the street whose hair you admire.

*

Pay a little extra to book the salon's master stylist. This is a stylist who has extra training and probably teaches or lectures.

*

If you are done in less than 30 minutes, move on. That's not enough time, and they're not customizing to your needs.

*

Enter the salon with a specific game plan (take a picture along if you need to, but try to be realistic).

## Use the Right Shampoo

There are very specific shampoos on the market today to help you make your hair be the best it can be.

*

Occasionally add a couple of caplets of vitamin E to your inexpensive shampoo for extra nourishment.

*

There are very good shampoos that perform more than one task.

*

Use inexpensive brands to strip off extra mousse, gels, etc., at least once a week.

## Condition When You Need To

You probably only need to deep condition (10 to 30 minutes) once or twice a week.

Your facial moisturizer can double as a hair conditioner in an emergency. Pat a small amount over dry hair.

If your hair is extremely dry, allow a little conditioner to remain in your hair. The excess will be rubbed off during the towel-drying process.

## The Grand Finish

Mousse is a good ending product for fine hair.

Gel is great for control, but should be used in very small amounts (about the size of a dime).

Hair spray should be used at least ten inches away from the sides of the head, and about five inches from the top.

Always use your fingers as a styling aid while using these products.

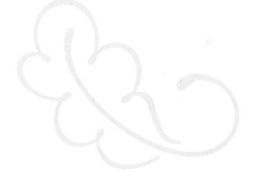

# Back to Nature

## Egg Shampoo

Beat 2 eggs in a cup of warm water. Massage the mixture into wet hair. Leave on for 5 to 10 minutes. Rinse in tepid water.

Caution: If you rinse in hot water, the eggs could scramble right in your hair and be impossible to get out!

## Lather and Strengthen

Mix an egg into your regular shampoo.

## To Thicken Hair

Add a tablespoon of powdered gelatin to your shampoo.

## Hair Shiners

1/4 cup lemon juice added to 1/2 cup water for light hair.

1/4 cup vinegar added to 1/2 cup water for brunettes.

Use as a final rinse.

## Conditioner for Dry Hair

Mix 1 egg, 1 teaspoon honey, and 2 teaspoons olive oil. Apply to wet hair. Cover with a shower cap or layer of plastic wrap. Leave on for at least 30 minutes before shampooing out.

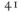

## Nourishing Hair Pack

Here's what to do with an overripe avocado:
Mash it up, and blend through dry hair. Leave the mixture on for 30 minutes. Shampoo thoroughly.

## Damaged Hair Repair

Mash a ripe banana and mix with a few drops of almond oil. Massage over entire head. Leave on for 15 minutes, then rinse thoroughly.

## Yogurt Conditioner

Use plain yogurt as a conditioner/final rinse.

Massage in after shampooing. Leave on 20 minutes. Rinse with warm water.

## Hot Oil Treatment

Mix 1 cup olive oil and 1/4 cup butter. Microwave for one minute. Leave on 20 minutes. Shampoo.

## Oily Hair Treatment

Add 1/4 cup aloe vera gel to 1/2 cup shampoo. Mix well and apply.

## Dry Hair Treatment

Mix 1 tablespoon honey to 2 tablespoons shampoo. Shampoo as usual.

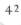

# Natural Color Enhancers

## Light Hair

Brew a cup of very strong chamomile tea. Let it cool to lukewarm. Spray or comb into dry hair. Leave on about 20 minutes. Shampoo and rinse.

This will give a color lift to blonde and light brown hair.

## Dark Hair

Brew an espresso or other strong coffee. Let it cool to lukewarm. Add to dry hair. Leave on 30 minutes. Then rinse thoroughly with tepid water.

This will add sparkling highlights to black or dark brown hair.

## Natural Styling

Flat beer is a cheap but effective styling tool. Pour a small amount in a spray mister (available at florist shops, hardware stores, and beauty supply centers). Spritz on before setting hair. Don't worry, the smell disappears when your hair dries. Beer will also give life to a tired perm or naturally curly hair that tends to droop. In this instance, you would spritz the beer on dry hair and scrunch the style into shape.

My beautiful colleagues who are also devout environmentalists swear to me that the following works better than any hair spray:

Dissolve a tablespoon of sugar into a glass of hot water. Allow it to cool, and use in a spray bottle.

# Rules for Highlighting Hair

1. Stick to gold or amber streaks if you have dark blonde or brown hair, and gold or strawberry streaks if you have auburn hair.

2. Don't place highlights too close together. Allow about an inch between.

3. To brighten your complexion, add a few subtle highlights to your bangs and along the sides of your face.

4. To make hair look thicker and fuller, brush highlights along the curves of your cut or on natural curls and waves.

5. To give the illusion of lighter hair, brush highlights throughout your hair, concentrating on your hairline, part, and bangs.

6. Bobs and layered cuts are best suited to highlighting.

7. Condition regularly, but avoid hot-oil treatments. They tend to strip color.

# Dandruff

Vitamin E capsules or vitamin E oil rubbed into your scalp will take away those ugly flakes.

Aloe vera gel applied all over your head will work immediately. Let it set for about 5 minutes, shampoo, and rinse.

I interviewed world-famous hairstylist to the stars, Dusty Fleming of Beverly Hills, who provided me with a unique dandruff shampoo:

Mash 30 aspirin tablets. Add to any bottle of shampoo. No need to refrigerate.

## Dry Cleaning

When shampooing is not an option, use either 2 tablespoons of cornstarch or 1 tablespoon of talcum powder and brush through the hair.

## tip

**A**ny strong dandruff shampoo will work in an emergency to remove extra color from chemically treated hair. Use it in a pinch when you leave your solution on too long.

## Coloring Tips

1. Women with pink complexions should avoid shades of red or golden blonde. Use ash tones to neutralize your coloring.

2. If your complexion is creamy white, pick dark shades (brown, black, or burgundy). They make the skin look luminous.

3. Sallow complexions should stay away from yellow, gold, or orange tones. Try deep reds and burgundies instead.

4. Starting at age forty, choose one shade lighter than your natural color.

5. Women of color should stay close to their natural hair color to complement the skin's tone.

## Hair Rules to Live By

1. The shorter your forehead, the longer your bangs should be. And they should start further back on your head.

2. Protect your hair, as well as your skin, from the sun. Use a sunscreen on hairline parts. Lip balm will also work since it contains a high SPF.

3. To completely remove residue from hair, combine equal amounts of baking soda and shampoo. Let set for five minutes.

4. Occasionally shampoo hair with mild dish washing detergent to get rid of product buildup.

5. Don't smile when the hairdresser is cutting your bangs.

Smiling raises your forehead, and your bangs might get cut too short.

6. Don't cross your legs during cutting. It will make you sit unevenly, and one side of your hair may end up longer than the other.

7. Don't try to style soaking-wet hair. Get it 80 percent dry first.

8. Hold your head upside down while drying for extra lift.

9. A vent brush will give your hair more volume.

10. Tease your hair with a toothbrush or baby comb. The small bristles will add a lot of volume to small sections of hair.

11. Use a ponytail to create an instant face-lift.

12. Reactivate a style by spritzing with spring water.

13. Never wash hair with hot water.

14. Always use a metal core brush to dry hair. The metal locks in heat to make hair dry faster, and tames and polishes hair by smoothing cuticles.

 tip

Take a strand test to make certain that you're using the correct shampoo for your hair type.

Does it snap easily? Your hair is fine or oily.

Is it hard to break? Your hair is coarse or dry.

# Hair Secrets

## Wet Hair Woes

Here's a way to leave the house with damp hair and style!

If hair is wet, run styling lotion or gel throughout. Spritz hair spray onto a brush and brush hair back, letting the sides curve down. Finish with more spray.

Never go to bed with wet hair! No, I'm not kidding!

What do mouthwash, fabric softener, and wine have to do with hair? They're unconventional hair treatments that *really* work! Read on!

## Red Wine

Neutralize the green color caused by chlorine by dabbing a little red wine onto the hair. Use it as a precaution before entering the pool. Use it before shampooing.

## Mouthwash

Mix 1/4 cup mouthwash with 1 cup water. Apply to scalp as a cleanser. Use after shampooing.

DO NOT RINSE OUT!

## Fabric Softener

The best leave-in conditioner is none other than laundry room fabric softener. It's very strong, so be sure to dilute it.

Suggestion: 1 cup water, 1/2 cup fabric softener.

Experiment with different softener scents for your own personal hair "signature." Save $$$$$ over expensive hair products!

## Women of Color

Jojoba oil slicks hair back beautifully!

Texture is key to controlling style.

Glover's Mange keeps black hair moist and encourages growth. You can find it at most beauty supply stores.

Conditioning is vital, as hair tends to be dry and brittle.

Copper and chestnut are good color options for warm or amber tones.

Don't blow dry hair too often. Let air dry whenever possible, and then blow it into style when it is just slightly damp.

A paddle brush is perfect for keeping hair at its most manageable.

Only allow the most experienced hands to handle weaves.

Women of color look great in hair colors of deep wine, red, or blue-black.

# Making Up

# *Making Up Is Not Hard to Do!*

Everyone has time to make their faces more attractive. Making time is the key to applying any cosmetic. The purpose of a beauty product should be to make the face look more lively, interesting, younger, prettier, or more polished. Making up your face means looking like *you*, but even better! This chapter is all you need to know to maximize your best assets while minimizing any defects. I'll show you how to do it whether you have 20 minutes or 20 seconds. You *do* have time to show your best face to the world.

# How Much Time Should You Spend on Your Makeup?

### 15 minutes?
### 10 minutes?
### 5 minutes?
### 2 minutes?

No matter where you're going, your usual routine should be no more than 15 minutes. The trick is to change your routine. There is no way that you can apply 15 minutes of cosmetics into a quick 5-minute regimen. You can still look pretty great in just a couple of minutes with my streamlined techniques. There's just no excuse for looking naked, tired, or "war-painted" anymore.

## Apply Makeup to a Clean Face

For best results, always start with a fresh face. Think of your face as a blank canvas. You are the artist, and you must start with a clean slate. Your makeup will go on more smoothly, more evenly, and last much longer.

# The Basics

## Foundation

A good foundation is the hardest-working cosmetic you will ever purchase. Choose one that is right for your skin type. An all-in-one foundation that gives adequate coverage is the combination liquid/powder duo found at every price level. I especially like the lower-cost lines found in Cover Girl, Revlon, and L'Oreal. They're less drying than the more expensive brands, and you don't have to wet them to get a flawless finish.

Do you look good in pure white? Look for "cool" shades.

Do you look better in cream or off-white? Choose "warm" tones.

Take a coral lipstick and a pink lipstick. If your skin more closely resembles the pink, you have pink undertones. The closer match to the coral means that you have a "yellow" undertone.

Now you can take this knowledge and confidently choose your own color at drugstores and mass-merchandise stores.

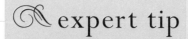

expert tip

To get the most out of your facial products, rub a small amount between your hands before applying. This action produces heat, making any cosmetic more spreadable.

I can't begin to tell you how many complaints I have heard from women who have been given the wrong color by those so-called "experts" behind the cosmetic counters. It's time for you to become your own expert. After all, who's been looking at that skin in every kind of light imaginable for all these years? Furthermore, if you make a mistake at the drugstore, it's easy to go back and get the next shade (lighter/darker) or even to blend the two at a far less exorbitant price.

# Eyebrows

The eyebrow is the frame of the face. It is easy to "lift" the eye with a couple of quick strokes. Many great beauties are known for their distinctive eyebrows (think Brooke Shields, Cindy Crawford, and Joan Crawford).

Control your eyebrows with an old toothbrush or an old washed mascara wand.

## WHICH TWEEZER?

*Thin Tip* — Good for grasping small, fine hairs and getting at ingrown hairs.

*Slanted Tip* — A versatile tweezer affording maximum control.

*Square Tip* — Best used for removing coarse hairs or several hairs at a time.

## MYTH: NEVER PLUCK ABOVE YOUR BROW.

Whoever thought of that one? You pluck where you need to pluck!

I once did a makeover on a woman who had these ugly hairs sticking up on her forehead. When I asked her why she didn't pluck them out, she recited to me this silly old outdated "don't touch those hairs above the eyebrow" rules.

## TECHNIQUE

Brush the brow upward and outward to define the natural line. Tweeze under the brow to form an arch. Soften the sting by rubbing the area with an ice cube. If you're completely clueless on what shape to make your eyebrow, cut out an eyebrow from a magazine, and stencil it on top of your own. Tweeze to trace the prototype.

## SECRETS OF EYEBROWS

Eyebrows look best when filled in with a soft pencil or powder. The modern brow is neither too thick nor too thin. Undecided? Go to a professional for your first plucking. It's most effective to work in bright natural light when tweezing. Soften the look of the brow by patting lightly with translucent powder. You can also substitute pale eye shadow to lighten a brow.

# Eyes

## APPLICATIONS

*Wide-set eyes*  To make your eyes look closer together, apply deep-toned shadow to the inner halves of the lids. Light-toned shadow goes on the outer halves.

*Closed-set eyes* Open up eyes by brushing deep-toned shadow on the outer half of the lids. Blend from the center of the eyes out and up to just above the crease. Use a light shadow on the inner halves of the lids and just under the brow bone.

## SECRETS

To make the whites of your eyes look brighter, use a light blue pencil under the eyes. Blue eye shadow lightly applied under the eyes works just as well.

Separate clumpy eye lashes with a lash comb available at beauty supply stores.

To get the best curl out of eyelashes, use a blow dryer

to heat an eyelash curler for about five seconds before using.

If you need to go from day to evening without starting from scratch, apply an eye foundation before shadowing.

Use waterproof formulations whenever possible.

Always wipe wands off before using to avoid clumping.

When applying mascara to bottom lashes, hold a tissue under the lash so that mascara doesn't end up on the skin.

Are you an absolute klutz when it comes to lining your eyes? Use a shadow as liner, or steady your hand by leaning your elbow on a table when applying.

# APPLYING FALSE EYELASHES

False eyelashes should be applied after foundation and eyebrows.

1. Powder eyelids.

2. Curl eyelashes to blend in with false ones.

3. Apply glue to lashes, being sure not to touch the lashes themselves.

4. Use a small stick (a toothpick works well) to be more precise.

5. Make sure that the lashes match by starting at the outer corner.

6. To blend false and natural lashes, apply a deep liquid liner over both.

## MORE SECRETS...

Make your eyeliner last each time you sharpen it by putting it in the freezer for at least 15 minutes prior to sharpening. This will ensure a perfect point with no crumbling.

Bend the tip of your mascara wand until it's angled to resemble a dentist's mirror. The wand will be easier to control, and the brush will give better coverage.

Pull your eyelid taut when applying eyeliner.

It actually helps to keep your mouth open when applying eye makeup. It keeps you from blinking.

Always apply liner in short, feathery brushes.

Neutral shadows are the most flattering to the eye.

Create a V-shape with a soft powder at the outer corner of the eyes to lift.

## Lips

Lipsticks have three basic components:
1. Pigment: Determines the color.

2. Emollients: Carry the pigment to the lips.

3. Waxes: Give the lipstick its shape. Choose the best formula!

## safety tips

Keep container lids and caps tightly closed.

Keep all applicators clean.

Store eye makeup at room temperature.

Don't let cosmetics sit on top of the radiator.

Use disposable products whenever possible.

Replace products often.

If a product produces an odor, toss it immediately.

Never rest an applicator on a public sink or vanity.

Never share your makeup.

Lipsticks also have three finishes:

1. Matte: The most lasting formulation. Not shiny. Flat coverage. (Caution: Pick one that's not too drying.)

2. Creamy: Looks best when first applied. Gives the most even coverage. Available in the widest array of colors.

3. Stain: Usually contains moisturizing ingredients. Gives only a hint of color. Wears off most naturally and discreetly. Most likely to have added sunscreen.

## SECRETS

For a softer lip color, blend moisturizer into the lipstick.

To change the color of any lipstick, lightly apply yellow eye shadow on the lips as a primer. This will warm up any color.

Blend lip liner and lipstick together on the back of the hand for a longer-lasting look.

If your lipstick tends to "bleed," apply lipstick first, then line over it to set.

Create your own lip colors by mixing different colors and textures of lipstick.

Right from the Experts!
To achieve a pouty, sexy mouth, emphasize your top lip by dabbing just a touch of gloss in the center.

To keep lipstick on while dining, keep lips off utensils. Use your lower teeth and tongue to do the work.

If you feel that your lips are unbalanced, use a lighter colored lipstick on the smaller lip.

A little bit of red or orange in the center of the lips makes them look fuller.

# Bronzing Powder

Ask any beauty what product she would most like to have on a deserted island, and the answer would most likely be her *bronzing powder*. This is the most versatile cosmetic you will ever own. Bronzing is the way to finish your face. Forget blush! I have never seen more beauty blunders than I have with the misuse of blush. I can't begin to tell you how many stripes and circles I have had to wipe off. Use blush improperly and you end up looking like a circus clown or a road marker. This is why I suggest (no, implore) you use bronzing powder to add color to your face. It's the perfect tool for nonprofessionals to use to contour their faces. Use it on the cheeks, down the sides of the nose (to slim), under the jawline (to take away a double chin or drooping jowls), and to add color to the face. You'll find bronzing powder readily available at drugstores, cosmetic counters—wherever your budget takes you. But please get some and use it! Why take risks with the sun when you can get a better sun-kissed look with this wonderful product? Can you tell it's my favorite all-time cosmetic?

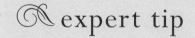 expert tip

Bronzer is absolutely elegant for creating a monochromatic look. Use it to shadow eyes, as a finishing powder for lips, to soften eyebrows, and as a finishing powder to set makeup. Don't go too dark. A shade or two darker than your regular color is best.

# Darker Skin Tones

Deeper complexions provide the perfect canvas for creating dramatic looks, but all products need to be carefully chosen and correctly applied to enhance the skin's unique tone and texture.

## Foundation

There are more than forty shades between the lightest and deepest of dark skin, so finding the right foundation can be a real challenge. Always test foundation on your cheek or jawline. The skin around the outside of the face is often darker than the skin in the center. Very dark skin has a lot of yellow pigment, so look for foundations with yellow undertones. Choose oil-free formulations, as darker skin reflects more light and is often slightly oily. Finish with a powder that's either transparent or slightly lighter than your skin.

## Eyes

The general rule is that the darker the skin, the deeper the eye color. This is because darker skin tends to absorb color. Use rich eye colors like gold, deep gray, purples, russet, copper, and brown. Pale pink and beige are enhancing highlighters. If your eyebrows are a little sparse, use dark brown or black pencil to fill them in. Use a kohl pencil to rim your eyes and a couple of coats of mascara.

## Lips

The same rule of "the darker the skin, the darker the color" applies to the lips. Red lips are perfect for evening, but choose reds with warm, brown tones, rather than blue undertones, which tend to be too cold. Women with darker tones usually have darker pigmentation outlining their lips, so they have their own natural lip line. If you do find that you require a lip liner, stay in the brown tones.

## Blush

Peach or brown tones are most flattering to darker skin. You'll find that pink shades contain too much of a blue undertone. For day wear, use a large soft brush to spread the color. For evening glamour, use a bronze shade a couple of tones darker than your natural skin color.

# The 15-Minute Face

Here's how to apply your makeup when you've got time to create a total look that can take you through the entire day.

1. Apply foundation with fingers or a sponge. When you're searching out a look that's more "natural," your fingers are the best makeup tool. The warmth of your fingers allows your foundation to spread quickly and more evenly. You'll also have more control. Start at the under-eye area. This is where coverage is needed the most. Blend all over the face, including lips. Sweep more heavily over flaws. Go lightly even over your "good" areas to even out the color.

2. To get a professional-looking eyebrow, follow these steps: Brush brows down, using a toothbrush or lash comb. Fill in with a soft pencil. Spray a toothbrush with hair spray. Brush brows back up and into place.

3. Two steps to beautiful eyes. Step One: Brush medium-toned shadow in a neutral shade over the entire lid. Deepen color in the crease and slightly above the outer corner of the eye, using a kohl pencil or darker shadow dipped in water. Smudge together to eliminate any unnatural looking lines.

Step Two: Lightly powder lashes to give mascara a coat to cling to. Line lids as close as possible with a pencil or liquid liner. Brush the first coat of mascara on. Comb through to separate hairs. Powder over liner in a shade just slightly lighter than the liner. Powder under eyes to complete the look.

4. Perfect lips. Use a neutral lip pencil rather than one that matches your lipstick. Apply lip pencil in dots around the lip, then play "connect the dots," following the natural lip line. Apply lipstick with a brush to make it last longer. After applying lipstick, pucker lips into an extreme "O." Cover your finger in a tissue, and poke it into your mouth. Twist away any excess color that could eventually end up on your teeth.

# The 5-Minute Face

To look completely set to go in five minutes or less, concentrate on the basics.

1. Apply foundation as a concealer on shadows and ruddiness.

2. Apply liner/shadow over and under lids.

3. Use a neutral lipstick on the apples of cheeks and lips.

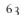

# The 2-Minute Face

1. Apply tinted moisturizer all over your face.

2. Sweep over a quick coat of mascara.

3. Apply bronzing gel on eyes, cheeks, and lips.

## Don't You Dare!

When you're in a rush, don't even try the following:

Liquid eyeliner: Needs time and a steady hand.

False eyelashes: Takes precision, strips, glue, and toothpicks.

Plucking: Takes time for the redness to disappear.

Lip liner: You could end up very uneven.

Foundation: Aim for a healthy glow instead.

# Double-Duty Cosmetics

Lipstick makes a great cream blush. You'll find it's a perfect way to color coordinate your face.

A nude pencil is just right to outline lips, cover blemishes, and line brows.

Eye shadow doubles as a lip powder.

Mascara can create an emergency beauty mark.

Dark brown eyeliner can be used as a lip pencil.

Dry blush can be used to seal lips or to change lip color. Or it can turn lip gloss into a longer-lasting, more matte formula.

Translucent powder can be used to lighten brows, seal lipstick, and to lighten dark areas.

Concealer hides redness and thins a too-prominent nose.

Powder puffs lightly sprayed with hair spray help powder stay put, and not on your clothes.

When retouching makeup in the middle of the day, go lightly. Oil from the skin will absorb the makeup's color and intensify it, making it look artificial. Press excess oil away with a tissue.

Pressed powder has a finer texture than loose powder, and looks less "floury."

Brush powder only on the center of the face. The sides of the face are always drier and don't require it.

# Models'
# Secrets

# *A Model's Bag*

A model's bag is filled with things you've never dreamed of! Here's a sampling of what you would find if you were to peek into the everyday bag of a working model.

P.S. Every model gets a workout just from lugging the thing around!

## Baby Wipes

This is a great tool for both cleansing the face and removing makeup. Baby wipes are hygienic (use them once and throw them away) and gentle to the face. You'll find that most versions contain lanolin, which is a skin softener. Purchase the convenient travel pack to freshen up at a moment's notice. It's also useful for taking up a stain or deodorant mark.

## Hemorrhoid Cream

As mentioned in chapter 2, it is the secret backstage of top runways. We use it on our puffy eyes, along the jawline, and on puffy cheeks. It is an instant face-lift, and a favorite of the die-hard partygoers.

## Garlic & Papaya Tablets

This is an absolute must when it's necessary to get weight off in a hurry. Garlic and papaya tablets act together as a diuretic and can get up to six pounds off in a couple of days. Ask your pharmacist for the strongest strength available over-the-counter. Take two garlic tablets with two papaya tablets before breakfast, lunch, and dinner. Eat lightly on these days, staying away from carbs and salt. There are "star" caplets out there on the market with similar ingredients priced at $100 and up. You can buy garlic and papaya tablets in your local drugstore or health food store. They're usually priced at under $5 each. Of course, being natural supplements, they're not as risky as the chemical weight-loss products so widely sold. However, don't take this increased dosage for more than two days.

## Chalk

Here's a natural way to hide stains. Carry white chalk for white clothing, and colored chalk for all the different colors of your wardrobe. I prefer that you use these natural treatments over chemical stain removers because they are safer for the planet and many fabrics can be ruined by chemical versions.

## White Eyeliner

Models find white eyeliner essential to create a wide-eyed look. Use it along the lash line, and softly smudge it with a sponge applicator. Use it inside the corners of your eye to open and widen.

## White Eye Shadow

Models use it to create a shimmering face base by mixing it with their foundation. Stroked just under the brow, it lifts the eye.

## Petroleum Jelly

You can create your own tinted gloss, and save lots of money at the same time. Simply mix any of your favorite lipsticks with a dab of petroleum jelly. You can also turn a powdered eye shadow into a glimmering eye shimmer with a drop of jelly.

## Eye Redness Reliever

Have I got a way for you to remove breakouts quickly! In just the way that an eye redness reliever takes the redness out of the eye, so does it remove redness from pimples. Squeeze out a little on a cotton swab. Hold it on the pimple for ten to fifteen seconds, or until it disappears. Models (and the people who hire them) consider it a catastrophe to get a pimple, but it's also important for you when you have that big party to obliterate the appearance of those little suckers. Anyone who has tried to mask pimples with makeup knows that it just doesn't work. This will do it, and quickly.

## Panty Hose

What do you think models do with ripped panty hose? They make their very own hair ties. You know, those fabulous hair accessories that pull your hair back with so much style, but cost a fortune? Here's what you do. Take the panty-hose leg (the more opaque styles provide more elasticity), and cut at two- to four-inch increments. You'll find that these hair ties will hold the hair beautifully with out any of the stress or split ends that rubber bands can cause. In addition, you can also use the color closest to your own hair color to make it blend.

## Erasers

What do models do when they lose an earring back? What do they do when their earring is just too heavy to stay properly on the ear? We take the eraser off a pencil and use it to hold that earring in place. Use this when you drop the back of an earring in your office, school, or at home. If you should find yourself in a restaurant, simply take a small piece of cork from your wine bottle.

# Hair Spray

Hair spray is helpful for keeping our do's in line, but it also prevents panty hose from running. Spray (lightly, please) a thin film up and down your hose before each wearing.

To keep your makeup in place, close your eyes and, holding the can at arm's length, spray a light mist of hair spray on your face. *Be very careful if you have sensitive skin!*

Should you happen to encounter an errant bug in your hotel room, just do what desperate yet resourceful models do. Take your hair spray and zap the pest with it. You will paralyze that little bugger more quickly than any insect spray ever did. Did you ever dream hair spray could be so versatile?

# Satin Pillowcase

A satin pillowcase is a model necessity. It keeps that hairstyle in place longer while traveling. Not only should you consider it an essential when you travel, but you'll also enjoy using it at home. Sleeping on a satin pillowcase will help prevent wrinkles while you sleep.

# Lemon Juice

Forget buying expensive toners. Models carry lemons in their bags to remove residue from their face and to refresh. The most diligent carry fresh lemons, but there's only so much one can stuff into those bags. If you do choose to purchase reconstituted lemon juice, make sure that it contains real lemon.

## Ice Water

You've heard that models drink lots of water. Well that's very true, but only half the story. To get optimum benefits from water, models drink ice water. With ice water, the body needs to use up to 30 calories just to warm itself to body temperature to absorb the water. You are actually using more calories than you are taking in.

## Teething Rings

Placed on the eyes, teething rings will reduce any puffiness, and provide a well-rested, wide-awake appearance. Frozen teething rings also soothe sunburned skin.

## Beef Jerky

Here is a snack that has been much maligned and is really quite good for staying lean. Turkey jerky contains less than one gram of fat, and has only 75 calories. What's especially appealing about turkey jerky is that it takes so long to chew (a good 20 minutes or so). This makes jerky orally gratifying. It may just keep you out of a few fast-food restaurants.

## Spoons

Here's yet another way to wake up tired eyes. Run a spoon under very cold water. Hold the spoon over the closed eye for about thirty seconds. The coolness of the metal "wakes up" the eyes.

## Parsley

Parsley is rich in chlorophyll. It is a major ingredient in leading breath fresheners, such as Clorets and Certs. Breath sweetening is more effective when it's done from inside the body. There is a lot of advertising going on now to get people to invest in internal breath fresheners. Again, don't spend a lot for these products. Do what knowledgeable models do to ensure "kissable" breath. Eat the parsley on your plate at mealtimes, or carry dried parsley in your bag to instantly freshen your breath. Parsley will keep your breath fresher a lot longer than topical fresheners will. Plus, it's healthy and low in calories.

## Tea

Tea helps keep cavities away! Both green and black tea contain fluoride and polyphenols to prevent plaque from adhering to the tooth's surface. Models drink tea for this very reason, and carry their tea bags faithfully. After models are done drinking their tea, they use their cooled tea bags to refresh their eyes. Simply squeeze the tea bag so that it isn't "dripping," and gently dab the bags under the eye area. If your face is clean, run over the entire face for a quick pick-me-up!

## Unfiltered Apple Cider Vinegar

What a versatile product! It's a great blood purifier when you add a tablespoon to a cup of hot water and drink it. You can also use it as an astringent for both your face and hair. Use it as a toner for your face and as a final hair rinse to remove residue.

## Avocado Body Butter

Models run to their nearest "natural" shop for this product. It gives a wonderfully smooth sheen to the skin. Even though it's a little bit sticky, it's very worthwhile.

## Toothbrush

Here's an old model's trick that everyone can copy. Brush your lips whenever you brush your teeth! Not only does it take away any chapping, but it plumps up the lip temporarily for that sought-after "pouty" look. A toothbrush is a super jewelry cleaner, getting into nooks and crannies, and it tames brows when lightly sprayed with styling gel.

## Tape

Models always carry double-sided tape to tack up fallen hems, make quick repairs to their clothing, and "quick tack" an accessory to clothing, hair, or purse.

## Candles

Carry a small birthday candle in your purse. Use it to get a stuck zipper going again.

## Colon Cleanser

No, I don't need to elaborate, but for beauty to really work, it needs to start from the inside.

Top actresses and great beauties throughout history have used this unconventional beauty/health regime. Legendary actress Mae West was famous for her daily enemas. Her skin was like silk until her death. These cleansers are now extremely popular, and expensive in spas. They are inexpensive and readily available at health food stores in kits and capsules.

## Jelly Beans

A jelly bean is a quick energy boost and surprisingly low in calories and fat. Most of these little treats contain only 5 or 6 calories each. Compared with a Lifesaver (10 calories) or stick of gum (up to 20 calories), it's a pretty good way to satisfy a sweet tooth.

## Kelp

Models carry kelp tablets to help speed up their metabolism. It should be available at your local drugstore.

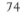

## Feverfew

Some super beauties eat feverfew sandwiches to relieve PMS and headaches. I would suggest that you get the tablets.

## Olive Oil

Here is an all-natural substance that models use on their hair when they're in the sun. Not only does it protect hair from the sun's harsh rays, but it becomes a deep-penetrating conditioner in the sun's natural heat.

## Rosemary Oil

Rubbed into the temple, rosemary oil relieves pain by relaxing constricted muscles.

## Candied Ginger

When traveling, models rely on candied ginger to prevent motion sickness.

## Dandelion Tea

This is used as a diuretic. Find this product in natural supermarkets and drugstores. Stay near a rest room!

# Brewer's Yeast

When a breakout occurs, it can sometimes mean the loss of an important job for a model. That's why models always keep brewer's yeast close at hand. Mixed with plain yogurt and applied to skin, it can prevent a pimple from coming through.

## Surgical Tape

Use surgical tape (available at most pharmacies) to smooth skin while you sleep. Tape an "X" between eyebrows, just above the nose. We often make many expressions while we sleep that can cause permanent wrinkling and furrowing.

## Lemon Peel

Lemon peel is a great natural mouthwash that is more effective than commercial brands. Combine the lemon peel with a small amount of witch hazel and rinse away.

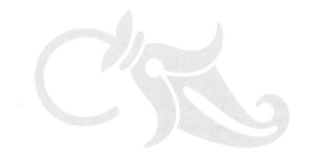

# How Models Get Great Skin

The following tips are from models who must remain anonymous because of contractual agreements.

"I drink a ton of spring water. I don't smoke, and I rarely drink. When I do drink wine, I always choose a spritzer. Before a shoot, I avoid fatty foods and chocolate."

"I boil some whole milk, then let it cool down. I lift off the film that forms on the surface, and apply it to my skin. After it dries, I scrub it off and exfoliate my skin."

"I wash my face with 2 teaspoons of sea salt, 1 tablespoon sesame oil, and 1/2 teaspoon lemon juice."

"I mash up a melon and leave it on my face for about 15 minutes. The melon is rich in beta carotene to combat cell damage."

"I add a tablespoon of honey to my bath. It invigorates my skin and leaves it feeling like silk."

# How Do Models Stay in Shape?

Sophie Dahl grows her own herbs and adds them to every dish to make low-calorie dishes more enjoyable.

Molly Sims swims and practices yoga daily.

Eva Herzigova starts every day with fruit and drinks different teas throughout the day.

# What Secret Do They Use Daily?

Alek Wek's skin is very dark and ashy, so she rubs baby oil all over her legs and arms at every photo shoot to give it glisten and shine.

Gisele Bundchen uses a dark concealer on the tip of her nose to make it appear shorter.

Naomi Campbell brushes her teeth, then makes sure to also thoroughly brush her lip area to keep it smooth and slightly plumped.

# Secrets of Taking a Great Picture

## Strike a Pose!

Years of taking pictures have yielded a list of dos and don'ts. Whether it's for a business picture, yearbook, or that special family event, make your next picture session an absolute success!

## What to Wear

Choose solid colors and avoid patterns, which grab too much attention away from the face.

Wear black and white with heavier emphasis on black for blondes and white for brunettes.

Avoid jewelry that would distract from the face or that would possibly date the photo.

Avoid clothing that would indicate a season or trend. Stay with classic clothing.

## Makeup

Don't use moisturizer under your foundation. It can look extremely "greasy" in a photo.

Use lots of powder, but make certain it's matte, not translucent.

If you'll be snapped by flash photography, go heavier on makeup. Flash photography bleaches out cosmetics.

Line lips, then dip a Q-tip in powder, and run along the line. This will create a mouth that "pops" out.

Never wear frosts or odd colors.

Avoid overstyling or "big" hair. It looks overdone.

Models prefer running to any other exercise. They choose it not only for their figures, but for healthy complexions.

Most models agree that on-the-job training is the only way to learn. Many of the most successful models never attended "modeling schools." Designers each have their own rules for walking the runway. Too much posing is out.

# Hands and Feet

# A Secret to None!

Now why would I devote an entire chapter to hands and feet? I can attest to the sabotage of a perfect look by the unkempt appearance of raggedy nails, uneven cuticles, and "never thought about it" feet (in sandals no less).

For those who have the time, it is really easy and fun to do your own manicure and pedicure. There are definite tricks to learn that will make you want to go the extra step, not to mention the savings. It's another canvas to paint.

# The 8-Step Perfect Manicure

## 1. File

Using an emery board, file nails straight up at the sides. Don't file sides of nails inward. The thinner your nail, the finer the emery board should be.

## 2. Cuticles

Apply cuticle softener to the edges of the nail. Massage gently with fingertips. If cuticles are very brittle, warm the softener in the microwave for a few seconds before applying.

## 3. Soak

Soak fingers in warm, soapy water. If fingers are discolored or dirty, take a tablet of denture cleanser and dissolve it in the water, or add a lime bleach.

## 4. Trim

Using a cuticle pusher/cutter (available at drugstores), push the cuticle back, and cut any excess hangnails. Don't cut in to your cuticle, because it will cause it to bleed.

## 5. Massage

Apply a moisturizer all over the hands, rubbing into the nails and cuticles. Distress by massaging the inside palm with your thumb.

## 6. Wipe

Dip a cotton ball in an astringent (like witch hazel or lemon juice), and remove any excess oil. This is necessary to allow polish to go on smoothly without bubbling.

## 7. Base Coat

Apply a base coat or primer, and allow to dry.

## 8. Final Coat

Brush on a one-coat polish. Look for the kind that contains both a color and top coat. It's just as good and a great time-saver.

# The Do-It-Yourself Pedicure

### 1.

Soak feet in shower gel or Epsom salts to soften.

### 2.

Separate toes with tissue.

### 3.

Apply non-acetone polish remover to eliminate oils.

### 4.

File to a square shape. Run the file vertically
over the nail to prevent future snags.

### 5.

Apply a base coat
(yes, this step is necessary even on a pedicure).

### 6.

Apply nail polish.

### 7.

Brush nails with oil to prevent ridges from forming.

### 8.

Allow polish to dry for 30 minutes.

# Special Problems

## Brittle Nails

Sun damage can cause brittle nails. Always apply sunscreen protection.

Once a week, apply an oil or cream and wear gloves on your hands overnight.

# Choosing a Nail File

One sure way to ruin your nails is by using the wrong nail file. There are files designed for artificial nails, files for buffing, and even files for both one-way and two-way filing. Here are some choices:

## Popsicle Stick File

This is the old standby. It's inexpensive and useful for natural nails.

## Metal File

It's a practical file that can be washed and reused. It will leave edges very smooth.

## Coarse File

This file has the texture of sandpaper and is best used on artificial nails.

## Two-Sided File

A practical file because of its dual purpose. The slightly abrasive side shapes natural nails. The smooth surface buffs and finishes them.

# Problems and Solutions

## Thickened Nail Polish

After you've stored nail polish for a while, it tends to thicken. Rather than toss it, turn the bottle upside down and roll it between your hands. Don't ever add nail polish remover to thin nail polish. Although it appears to thin it out temporarily, it will eventually dry the polish out and spoil whatever is left. When polish gets so gloppy that the colors separate, it's too old to keep. Get rid of it.

## Chapped Hands

Dry, chapped hands are a real problem to anyone who enjoys the outdoors or does heavy house-

work. One solution is to use a thick cream or salve. Many perfectly polished beauties swear by traditional petroleum jelly as a protectant. I find it a little greasy, but it is *great* as an overnight treatment under cotton gloves.

## Chipped Polish

Use a file and smooth out the chipped polish until the ridge is even with the nail. Apply polish only to the chipped area, and allow it to dry. Recoat the entire nail.

## Split Nail

Apply quick-drying glue to the split, and let dry. Smooth with a file or buffer. Mend with a tea bag by cutting a tiny piece from the tea bag. Cover the split, and dot on nail glue. Let dry and smooth with a buffer.

## Smudges

Apply polish remover to smudged polish to smooth out. Let it dry, and follow up with a thin coat of polish.

## Yellowed Nails

To prevent the discoloration that occurs with nail polish stains, always use a base coat of superior quality.

## Pale Nails

Although pale nails can be hereditary, it can also be the result of poor circulation or anemia. Take an iron supplement or add iron-rich foods to your diet.

## Peeling Nails

Avoid quick-dry polishes that contain acetone, which can dry out your nails. Always file nails lightly, just enough to shape and keep the layers even. Uneven nails have a tendency to peel.

## Brittle Nails

Moisturize with an oil or emollient. There are several on the market, but a vitamin E capsule works just as well.

## Artificial Nails

Although artificial nails can make your hands look more attractive, they can seriously damage your natural nail bed. The worst offenders are the glue-on variety, which cause some of the nail surface to get torn away when they are removed. Another problem is the glue, which can cause an allergic reaction. Pre-glued nails are less damaging, but last only three days.

## Foot Calluses

Always use a pumice stone. Razors and other cutters are now illegal for pedicurists to use.

## Cracked Hands

Better than lotion, mashed potatoes will solve this frequent problem. Boil a small peeled potato until soft. Mash with 1 tablespoon olive oil. Apply to hands and leave on for 15 minutes. Rinse with cool water.

## Aching Feet

Practice picking up small objects like marbles or tiny balls with your toes. Curl toes under, and hold that position for a few seconds. Repeat several times. Alternate walking on toes (like a ballerina) and heels every day.

# Insider Tips

Let fingers rest at least a day between manicures. This allows the nail a chance to "breathe."

Add 1/2 teaspoon of sugar to a dollop of hand cream, and massage the entire hand. This smoothes and softens.

Use an old eyeliner brush dipped in nail polish remover to clean up your manicure. Cotton swabs are too messy.

Always wash hands thoroughly before a manicure. If it's necessary to clean hands after nails are done, use a cleansing pad. Soap and water washes away protective creams left over from the manicure.

Use a face mask to treat your hands and feet. Hydrating masks work especially well. Gently file nails every other day to keep tips smooth and prevent snags and breaking.

# Secrets
## of Styling

# What Is Fashion?

Here's what you need to know. Style is not fashion, and fashion is not style. You can wear every trend that's come around the fashion bend in the last century and never be stylish. Conversely, you can scoff as fashions come and go and still be the doyen of style and good taste. Fashion changes by the minute, and we cannot take it too seriously. Caring too much is a sure sign of becoming a fashion victim. The majority of stylish women I have come across treat fashion with a degree of irreverence. You should too. Trust me, fashion is not and never has been brain surgery.

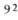

# What Is Style?
# It's Not Being Afraid to Stand Out!

Women of style are not afraid to take fashion risks. They are the ones who will take an article of clothing and wear it in a way it was never intended to be worn. For instance, it's the woman who will wear a classic pantsuit (maybe it's Armani) and accompany it with a campy T-shirt from her latest vacation. It's called "high-low" in the industry.

## Style Is Having a Trademark and Being Recognized for It

It could be something as simple as not being seen without that great black jacket. Or maybe it's that brown suede pant that looks chic and appropriate dressed up or down.

## Style Is Not Obeying Silly Fashion Rules

Okay, maybe you just love animal prints. You covet them whether or not they are on the fashion runways. You have dug through many thrift shop bins to add to your collection. Wearing these prints make you feel different daring, and alive. Style is having the good sense not to wear more than one piece at a time. Style is also knowing not to wear these pieces to a job interview or to a funeral. Get my point? That is style.

## Style Is Knowing When to Stop

The difference between stylish and tacky is wearing one, maybe two pieces, at a time. The secret to being well dressed is underdressing. This allows you to wear distinctive clothing that makes its own statement.

## Style Is Good Fit

Having a good eye for how clothing falls is key to looking just right. You need to know where those pants should fall and how that jacket must hang to flatter. It does no good to wear only the top designer names if the fit's not right. You can't be married to one size since each designer sizes differently. Try it on!

## The Classics

How do you define classic dressing? It is the backbone of fashion. It is what allows a woman to remain chic through every season of her life. These women, although not devoted to each year's runway trend, still look current and absolutely up to date.

Although their interest in fashion is ongoing, they're not obsessed, and they don't allow fashion to define who they are or what message they wish to convey.

> style is going with what works for you

If it feels comfortable, then you're going to get a lot more wear out of it. This is a fundamental concept of style that you should live with every single day. Even though it's right off the runway, unless you feel confident in it, leave it alone—especially if you find yourself pulling and tugging at it.

Classic dressers stimulate our own interest in appearance. They give us ideas, and they're meant to be noticed, much in the same way we admire art. But even the fashion magazines that display the latest and greatest don't want their pages to be taken literally.

Editors want you to look, admire, and then see how you can incorporate what you see into your own scenario. It is possible to bring the runway into real life with the right approach.

## A Classic Wardrobe

Here is my list of classic "must-haves." These are the things that you can keep twenty or thirty years, with only occasional updates for breakage, change of size, or just "weariness."

The sheath dress (goes under any jacket)

Gold hoop earrings or "diamond" studs

Black skirt

Tank top

Well-cut jacket

Basic trousers

White cotton shirt

A watch that can double as a bracelet

Black or white T-shirt

Cardigan sweater

Classic sunglasses

# Fashion Don'ts

Here is the ultimate list of a "never stylish" fashion victim. I don't care who wears them, how great a buy, or how great it makes them feel. Stay away!

- Lace or fishnet hose
- Sequins during daylight hours
- More than two theme pieces (western, menswear, alternative)
- Over-the-top pants
- Baby-doll dresses after high school
- A skirt shorter than eighteen inches
- Huge shoulder pads
- Sequined sweatshirts
- Jogging suits when you're not jogging
- Dirty sneakers
- Cheap fabrics
- Shoe heels higher than three inches
- More than two bracelets
- More than two earrings in each ear
- Transparent clothing
- Underwear as outerwear
- Ankle bracelets
- Acid-washed clothing
- Peter Pan collars
- Hats or sunglasses indoors
- Bra tops
- Belly buttons off the beach
- Clogs with skirts
- Tie-dye
- Madras

# Camouflage Dressing

No matter what size, age, height, or weight you are, you can look younger, thinner, and better than ever with the techniques I use when I'm doing makeovers and transformations. When I'm asked to do a TV makeover, invariably the producers ask me not to have the "transformee" appear ten pounds thinner, but hey, let's go for twenty pounds thinner. When TV ratings are on the sleeve, I have my work cut out for me, and I'd better deliver. Here are my tried-and-true secrets for camouflage dressing that I know will work for you.

After utilizing these tips, you will be assured by your own transformation that not all those gorgeous creatures you see in magazines, TV, and movies are anorexic, attached to their treadmills, or creatures from another planet. They are just real people, who know how to accentuate their own positives and downplay their negatives.

## Dressing Thinner

1. Match your hose to your shoes. Legs look longer and thinner when hose is toned to skirts and shoes.

2. An A-line skirt emphasizes body length while hiding thighs.

3. Use a shirt like a jacket or a tunic. Choose a generously cut shirt in a heavy or lined fabric. It's an elegant look over slim pants, flowing gently over every possible sin.

4. Dress in one color. Wearing one color from shoulder to shoe streamlines the body. It's called monochromatic dressing. If you don't want to limit yourself to just one color, choose dark colors that are closely matched.

5. If you have a chubby neck, choose v-necklines. They create the illusion of a longer, leaner body.

6. To bring attention to the face and away from the body, wear a pendant and matching earrings.

7. A long jacket is a "pound-parer." It can make any outfit look elegant while hiding figure flaws.

8. Choose a low-heeled shoe that is cut low on the instep. Stick to a thinner, more graceful heel.

9. Wear belts in a low slung manner or gently held around the waist.

10. Always wear control-top panty hose with Lycra.

11. Choose a slightly fitted jacket. A look that is too loose or boxy tends to add pounds.

12. Simple styling is most slimming. Cuffs, pockets, and buttons add width to the body.

13. Look for fabrics that drape the body. This would include light wool, cotton, and rayon.

## How to Spot a Fashion Victim

1. They buy clothes that they have no intention of wearing.

2. They purchase things without first trying them on.

3. They find things in the back of their closet, with the tickets still attached.

4. They purchase items that have nothing to do with their lifestyle, just because it's the latest trend.

5. They always look uncomfortable in their own skin.

# Good Jeans

Many of us feel that landing the perfect pair of jeans is much like finding a soul mate.

There really is something to be said for a great pair of jeans. Some women use them like a scale. They feel they're in shape when their jeans fit.

## How to Shop

### DON'T LET YOUR BODY TYPE LIMIT YOU

Anyone can wear jeans if they try on enough styles. Bring them all in and be patient until you find the one that works for you.

### DON'T BE AFRAID TO SHOW YOUR BODY

If you have an area that you're self-conscious to show, hiding it under pockets or baggy fabric is not your option. In the case of jeans, tighter can be more flattering.

### YOU DESERVE COMPLETE COMFORT

Make sure that you feel good in your jeans. There's a sense of sexy freedom that lends itself to jeans, unlike anything else when you're happy in them.

### DRESS UP YOUR JEANS

Jeans provide many options. Heels are fun, and silk sends your jeans to a party!

## LOOK AROUND

Check out magazines and celebrity pictures. If you see someone with a body similar to yours, then search those jeans out.

# Here's What to Like About Jeans

Jeans are classless.
No one can tell how much money
you have by your jeans.

Jeans are sexy.
If you get that just-right fit,
they can be sexier than lingerie.

Jeans are versatile.
There's almost no place that you can't wear jeans—
with the right finishing touches.

Jeans stand on their own.
All you need to do is add the right shirt or jacket
to look finished.

# Coats

Coats and jackets are frosting on the cake. It is one of the first things people see, and can be the core of a wardrobe. Don't wear an old torn coat if you can afford to change to a newer, fresher version. The abundance of cuts, colors, and fabrics means that there is the perfect coat waiting out there for you.

## Look for a Good Cut

You need enough room in the shoulder, sleeves, and torso to be comfortable.

## Durability

Look for sturdy lining. You'll find that the combination of rayon-acetate lasts the longest. Check to see that the lining is tacked down at appropriate locations. It should be attached at the cuffs, arm holes, and hem.

## Timeless Styles

Pea coat

Wrap coat

Princess shape

Military coat

Trench

Traditional camel

## Proper Length

Where do you most like to wear your hemlines? Make sure your coat covers the length you are most apt to wear. Best bet? Pick a coat that almost sweeps to the ankles. This coat will get you out the door with some dignity no matter what you have on underneath.

# Rules for Wearing Florals

1. Florals can never be a head-to-toe look. Choose your spot. A little goes a long way.

2. If you don't feel comfortable wearing florals, consider accessorizing with them. Try a scarf, floral mules, or a floral purse.

3. Never wear floral with black or other dark colors. Choose the palest hue in the pattern.

# Casual Chic

Casual chic is an easy and fun way to dress. Most days we are given the challenge of coming up with this style. The key is to appear like you arrived at your look with little or no effort.

## What's Not Casually Chic

Sweats

Anything too matched

Clothes that are uncomfortable

Anything overly tailored

Little-girl looks

Too many rips and tears

Stained clothing

Hose runs

Fallen hems

Worn-down shoes

Obviously cheap fabric

Too much jewelry

Too much perfume

Excessive makeup

Tight-fitting clothing

Un-ironed clothing

Lines or bulges under clothing

Pants that are too short

Pants that hit the pavement

Heels with shorts

Stirrups

Wedgies

Anything transparent without a camisole

# Swimwear

## Primal Fear

I have heard more screaming coming out of dressing rooms at swimsuit time than at any other time of the year. It doesn't matter what size you are or what age. Trying on swimwear has to rate right up there with the stirrups in doctor's offices. I'm not saying that purchasing a swimsuit will ever be enjoyable, but I can make it a little less painful for you.

## Rule #1—Go Up a Size

This is not what most women want to hear, but because swimsuits are made of less fabric than other garments, they tend to run a bit smaller than regular street clothing. A size-twelve suit will be very snug on a woman who wears a size-twelve dress, but will be perfect on a woman who wears a size ten. If you insist on trying on your regular size, be certain that you can bend, stretch, sit, etc., without any discomfort or riding up.

## Rule #2—Look at Tags

Thank the designer gods for finally listening to us. They have developed swimwear that actually gives off the illusion of having lost ten pounds. You'll see the features written right on the tag. Lycra is a good indicator that these suits are minimizers. Again, try them on, because you might find them quite confining. It's nice to be tucked in, but who wants to feel like they're wearing a girdle on the beach?

## Rule #3—Don't Be Afraid of Color

There is no reason to stick to black or navy if you're trying to give off the illusion of being slim. Although darker colors do make the body appear slimmer, vibrant shades like purple, magenta, maroon, and green also serve this purpose. You can effectively use color to accentuate the positives, while hiding any negatives. For instance, if you want to show off great legs, choose a bright skirt with a darker top. Don't be afraid of pattern or texture in the fabric. Vertical lines can be especially flattering, because people's eyes never rest on a specific body area. Patterns keep the eyes moving.

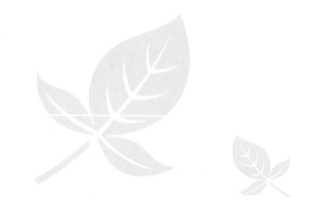

## Caring for Your Swimsuit

- Hand wash after every wearing.
- Never put your suit in the dryer.
- Always dry your swimsuit thoroughly before storing it.
- Try not to get any lotions or sunscreens on your suit.
- If you do get any creams on your suit, use shampoo to sponge it off.

# Working Style

## Dressing for Success

We all know about dressing for corporate climbing and how the image that you present at work can enhance your chances of promotion and/or a salary increase. But that's not all there is to that story. Just putting on any structured suit will no longer do. Your suit sends out a distinct message. The trick is dressing for the position you want and finding that fine balance between fitting in as a team member without sacrificing individuality. Many companies now realize that creative dressers are more open to new ideas than those who dress conservatively. How do you find the style that's right for you without being too risky? One that suits your body shape? Here are the secrets of a successful working wardrobe.

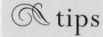 tips

1. The higher the quality, the better your suit will look in six months.

2. Buy a suit in a medium-weight fabric for year-round wear.

3. A neutral color will provide more flexibility to mix and match with other clothes in your wardrobe.

4. Single-breasted jackets are more slimming.

5. Vertical stripes make you look taller and slimmer.

# Choose a Style That Flatters Your Body Type

## TRIANGLE

Keep your jacket simple, yet slightly curvy.

## PEAR

Choose jackets with small, soft shoulder pads to give you more shape on top. Stay away from double-breasted jackets so that you don't add bulk to your hips.

## STRAIGHT

Give the illusion of a slimmer waist with a light-colored, loosely tailored jacket. Wear it over a fitted dark top and a belt.

## HOURGLASS

Sharp, masculine tailoring is not for you. Go for soft shapes and fabrics. You can get away with a knee-length pencil skirt or well-tailored trousers.

# How to Wear Pants

## Traditional

A flat-front straight-leg style is the most flattering for every body.

## Petite

Choose high-waisted styles to give off the illusion of a longer leg.

## Thin

Pleated trousers (menswear) creates a curvier leg.

## Full Tummy

Softly draped pants fall gracefully on the body.

# Shopping Secrets

## Try It On

Make sure you look great from all angles of the mirror.

## Stick to a List

Stay with the pieces that will fill out your wardrobe, no matter how great a "deal" it seems, or how trendy it is.

## Don't Wait Until the Last Minute to Shop

Never shop the day before an event. You are bound to make a big mistake. Of course, those last-minute events do occasionally occur. Just be prepared with a basic outfit that needs only the right accessories.

## Be Very Careful of Sales

It's only a good buy if you would have paid full price for it.

## Always Dress Well, and Wear Makeup when Shopping

This is so important, because if you have no makeup on, everything looks horrible. If you're not well dressed, even the lowly of the low looks better than what you have on.

## Shop Alone

Well-meaning friends can talk you into a less than flattering look (the "go ahead, you deserve it" routine), and salespeople can be just plain annoying. When one of them starts following you around the store, simply explain that you need to be alone to sort through your wardrobe needs. It works every time!

## Buy for the Body You Have

"It would look great if I just lost five pounds." How many of those promises do you have hanging in your closet? By the time you've lost the weight, that adorable outfit will be unfashionably out of style.

# Shopping Dos and Don'ts

## Do...

- Start your shopping trip in your own closet.
- Wear color near your face.
- Raid your man's closet.
- Choose your undergarments carefully.
- Wear white in winter. It's called winter white.
- Add a trendy touch to each season's wardrobe.
- Shop in resale shops.
- Keep a core of five or six basics in your wardrobe.
- Pick out two or three colors and plan your wardrobe around them.
- Develop a theme to your wardrobe.
- Purchase items that can be worn in any season.

## Don't...

- Be afraid to split up outfits.
- Overaccessorize.
- Try to hide figure flaws in oversized clothing.
- Wear tops that display your favorite beer, cause, pet, or political party.
- Wear a full jacket with a full skirt.
- Use more than two colors in an outfit.
- Wear linen in winter.
- Fix any part of your clothing in public.
- Overspend on an item that you don't really love.
- Send the wrong message with your clothing.
- Keep your clothes so plain that you fade into the woodwork.
- Purchase anything that requires time-consuming maintenance.

# chapter eight

# Glamour

# How to Go from Day to Evening

## Fashion Situation

The phone rings. The invitation comes. You are invited to that special event, but there's a real problem—there will be no time to change into evening attire.

## Solution #1

Wear a basic black dress, basic skirt and top, or well-cut trouser suit. Carry a few well-chosen accessories and stronger makeup colors.

## Solution #2

A classic white shirt can go right into evening with a frilly skirt and rhinestone accessories.

## Solution #3

A well-cut pair of trousers can take on a new life with a silk, embroidered, or sequined top.

## Solution #4

A basic black top can be belted with a rhinestone belt or ribbon and added to a satin skirt for last-minute panache.

## Solution #5

A basic suit jacket can go into the evening when paired with satin or lace slacks.

## Solution #6

Take a regular day suit, and remove the blouse under the jacket. Extra skin is appropriate for the evening hours. If you're feeling just too underdressed, then add a little lace hanky at the bodice.

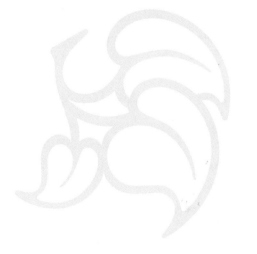

# What Does That Invitation Mean?

The invitation came in the mail today, and you haven't a clue what to wear. You've never been to this kind of event, and you won't know a soul there. Just what does this invitation mean?

## The Invitation Says *Informal*

Choose a classic look such as a sweater with flowing pants or a silk blouse with matching silk pants. Appropriate heels for the event would be in the two- to three-inch range. Flats won't make it here. Keep accessories toned down.

## The Invitation Says *City Attire*

Of course, this party or event would be taking place in or near a city. For this event, black is always safe. A black trouser suit would be perfect. Heels can be one to two and a half inches in height.

## The Invitation Says *Business / Cocktail*

Here's where that little black dress we all have in our closet comes in handy. Add a jacket according to your comfort level. You can always take it off should you find that the look is a bit too corporate.

## The Invitation Says *Formal*

This is the invitation that drives every woman crazy! What does formal really mean? When you receive this invitation, pull out that long dress or skirt. Mid-calf is only appropriate if the dress is very elaborate.

## Short or Long?

A long formal gown is limiting. When in doubt? Go for short. And don't forget—extra glamour means extra makeup.

## The Invitation Says *Black Tie*

When black tie is required, think formal but understated. You can show up in a long dress, but a well-fitted dress and jacket would be just as acceptable. A satin dress or tuxedo pantsuit is perfectly fine.

# What to Wear to a Wedding

## Pants

A pantsuit is always chic. Make certain it's in a dressy fabric.

## Black

Although black is acceptable, navy is much more modern.

## White

Don't wear it, and I don't care what the etiquette experts say. Beige is more flattering and more respectful of the bride.

## Sequins

Don't wear any unless the wedding starts at 6 p.m.

# Hair

## Instant Glamour

To give hair fullness and bounce, lift dry hair at the roots with a round brush. Pull it taut, and spritz with hair spray. Then blow-dry hair on the warm setting at high heat. Using the warm setting makes hair flexible and allows you to restyle it. For even more fullness, bend forward so that head is tilted down when drying. Finish styling as usual.

## Sparkling, Shining Hair

Give your hair a dazzling, party-perfect finish by spritzing it with a shine spray. There are several good ones on the market. Apply shine through dry hair, then brush through for even distribution. Ionic hair dryers and flat irons will help increase shine.

# Eyes

## Fast Frames

To give the eye definition, brush brows up to accentuate the arch. Set brows with a toothbrush sprayed with hair spray. Finish by adding a bit of white shadow under the brow. If necessary, before spraying, pencil along the natural arch.

## Mystery Eyes

The smoky eye is the perfect look for "after five." Take a black pencil or liquid liner, and line both above and below the eye. Soften and secure the look by running over the lines with a similar-colored shadow.

# Take the Plunge

Slinky, low-cut dresses put it all out there! Make sure your skin is blemish-free by gently exfoliating to lift off dead skin, even out skin tone, and discourage breakouts. Toners will help keep oiliness under control, so be certain to wipe off residue with witch hazel or lemon.

If you do have blemished skin, don't panic! Take a water-resistant concealer, and pat it over the area until it blends with the surrounding area. A quick pat of powder will set it. If you have lines, smooth a firming face gel over the area (be sure to check the breast area).

Keep skin soft and silky by spraying on body oils that both scent and polish shoulders, breasts, and upper arms. Here's a way to boost the sheen. Just mix a touch of gold powder with the oil in the palms of your hands, then smooth it on.

Add a little bronzing powder into the cleavage, but be sure to blend well.

# The Evening Bag

There are two schools of thought when it comes to evening bags. There's the person who carries as little as possible, and then there's the person who can't go out for the evening without throwing in the kitchen sink. There are guidelines for both; just plan ahead!

## The Minimalist

### MONEY?
Enough cash to hail a cab

### COSMETICS?
A lipstick and compact

### ANYTHING ELSE?
Breath mints
A comb
A driver's license
Maybe a hanky

## The Pack Rat

### MONEY?
Not only a substantial amount of money (up to $100), but a credit card (or two)

### COSMETICS?
Lipstick, foundation, blush, mascara, and liner
Superglue to tack back false eyelashes

### ANYTHING ELSE?
Cell phone
Tampon
Key
Business cards

# The Finishing Touch

# Didn't You Know?

## Accessories Make the Woman

Show me a well-dressed woman, and I'll show you someone who has mastered the fine art of accessorizing. Accessories are the finishing touch that gives us our individuality and shows us how far we can take a look with a little imagination. It is the least expensive way to extend a wardrobe and the first evidence of good taste. Here's what I consider to be the most important accessories in any woman's wardrobe.

## The Handbag

You thought shoes were the most important accessory in a woman's wardrobe? Wrong! It's your handbag...your purse...your pocketbook. It's at eye level after all! The perfect handbag is never larger than 10 x 13 inches. Although it's not necessary to match a handbag to every outfit, there should be some kind of coordination effort. Always choose the best handbag you can possibly afford. To be well-groomed, it is absolutely essential for you to include the following items.

## THE ESSENTIALS

Lipstick (doubles as blush)

Compact (choose dual finish)

Notebook with pen

Wallet

Breath mints

Comb or brush

Neutral eye shadow (doubles as lip powder)

Eyeliner

Tissues

## IF THERE'S STILL ROOM, ADD THESE

Mini pill box with supplies

Sewing kit

Mascara

Hair elastic

Nail file

# While on the Go

## Time-Savers

Carry your makeup in a see-through pencil case. It will eliminate wasted time rummaging through your entire bag, ruining your manicure.

Always carry a mirror in your bag.

Don't ever carry loose powder!

If you must choose one color, pick a neutral bag, which will go with about everything!

Be sure that the handles fit neatly over your shoulder before purchasing your bag. A handbag, while trendy, is impractical for daily use.

# Shoes

I have never had a problem convincing women of the importance of shoes. It's the men who wear their shoes forever, and get them soled and resoled like they're desperate to keep an old friend. It's the type of shoe that women choose that can make or break a totally finished look. Also, the care they give their shoes is key in giving that all-important finishing touch. Scuffed heels, sloppy fit, and salt marks can be fixed in moments. As well they should!

## Heels

Allow me to share an old model's trick with you. A lot of modeling is not as glamorous as you may have been led to believe. There are levels of modeling that include promotion work, trade shows, and other similar assignments. It means that these beautiful models must remain on their feet, in high heels, and looking glamorous for hours at a time.

How do they do it without collapsing? The secret is to go up one full size from your regular shoe size. If you're a size 8 in a loafer, then you would take a size 9 in a three-inch heel. This allows for the inevitable swelling that takes place during the day. For those who need to look "together" and polished throughout a long and tedious workday, heels from one and a half to two inches high are the most comfortable. Also, don't overlook comfort inserts available at drugstores.

# Fabric

If you can afford the rich, buttery leather of a designer shoe, your benefits include comfort and flexibility. If it's completely out of your price range, try to stay away from heavy, man-made materials. They don't last very long, and they are low on the comfort scale. It's impossible for a foot to breathe in vinyl or plastic.

Shoes that are tight when you are being fitted will never become comfortable. The one exception is suede, which does tend to stretch after wearing.

Perhaps you have those shoes that you just couldn't resist—the ones that you hoped would stretch out—sitting in your closet. Try this: Wet the inside of the shoes with an equal amount of water and alcohol. Stuff the shoes with newspaper, and leave them out to dry overnight. This just might make them wearable.

# What Else to Watch Out For

## BACK HEIGHT AND HEEL PINCH

Hold backs together to check that they are equal height. Then put each shoe down to make sure that they sit flat.

## TOE SPRING

You should be able to slip a pencil under the front of the shoe.

## SYNTHETICS/LEATHER

The label should state clearly what the shoe is made of.

## TOP LINE

Look at the inside of the heel to check that the shoe's outside rim is straight.

## TOPSTITCHING

This should be straight and well-machined. If it's uneven, the shoe is poorly made.

## SOLE BONDING

If you can pull the insole away, they haven't used the right adhesive. Under the inner sole, you should have a little cushion for comfort.

## HEEL ATTACHMENT

If you run your finger around the inner sole and feel bumps, the wrong kind of nail has been used.

## STITCHED SOLE

A leather sole should be stitched (or welted) to the upper sole. A channel is cut into the sole, the shoe is stitched together, and then the channel is put back to hide the stitching. You should clearly see the welt mark running all around the sole. Leather soles are better than resin.

# Sandals

1. Consider what you'll be wearing with your sandals, and purchase the simplest pair.

2. If you tend to wear patterns, choose black or neutral sandals.

3. Buy the right size. Your heels and toes should not hang over the edges of the sandals. Make sure that the strappy parts of the sandals aren't too tight or flimsy.

# Hosiery

The purpose of everything I share with you is meant to simplify your life, not complicate it. That is why I refuse to go into a long soliloquy on what percent of nylon versus Lycra you should have in your hose for longevity. Here's are the rules. Follow them, and you'll get the most bang for your buck.

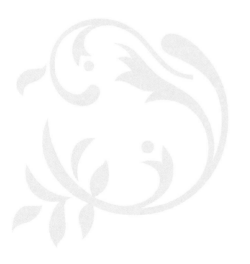

## Do...

Wear black opaque stockings. They are the most practical and slimming hose you'll ever own.

Match your shoes and hose when you can. This is a very appealing and slimming look.

Hand wash your hose in a mild detergent.

Use reinforced toes when not wearing open-toed shoes.

Stock up on your favorite hose when they go on sale.

Give your hose a quick spray of hair lacquer to resist runs.

# Sunglasses

Another important finishing touch to any woman's wardrobe are sunglasses. The general rule is to choose a frame that complements your facial structure.

## Long, Narrow Face

Looks best in wraparound oval frames.

## Round Face

Looks best in square glasses.

## Square Face

Looks best in round frames.

## Long Nose

Stay away from aviator styles.

# Jewelry at Work

Don't be afraid to show your personal style at work. It can add sparkle and fun to an otherwise serious environment.

The right jewelry can make whatever you wear more sophisticated and noteworthy. Keep jewelry understated in the workplace. Bracelets shouldn't get in the way of writing or typing. While one or two conversation pins are a statement, several pins become a walking jewelry chest.

# Jewelry Dos and Don'ts

## Do...

- Mix metals.
- Mix pearls with metals.
- Pile on several chains together (this look was invented by Coco Chanel).
- Bring daytime into evening with crystal jewelry.
- Be creative with your jewelry. Wear it on a purse, at your waist, or even on your watch.
- Combine short chokers with long strands.
- Use bracelets to create cuffs.
- Use unusual pins as icebreakers at an event where you're not known.

- Use a pin as a necklace enhancer to change a look.
- Tack down a scarf with a coordinating pin.
- Dress up denim with jewelry.
- Soften the look of leather with pearls.
- Use power jewelry for evening.
- Bring a trouser suit into evening with crystal pieces.
- Feel free to knot double and triple pearls.
- Add two chokers at once (a wonderful frame for the face).
- Mix real gems with fake.
- Mix matte and shiny materials.

# Don't...

- Wear dangle jewelry at work.
- Wear perfume near pearls (the oil will eat away the coating).
- Wear jewelry in your nose.
- Wear big earrings and a big necklace.
- Wear a lot of crystal or sparkle during the day.
- Wear white jewelry with white clothing.
- Wear a daytime watch with evening attire.
- Put a dainty ring on a large hand.
- Be afraid to wear heirlooms.

- Think of costume jewelry as tacky.
- Wear pendants longer than the belt line.
- Forget to coordinate your jewelry with your belt (both are important accessories).
- Be afraid to wear a pin or two on your shoulder to pick up your posture.
- Wear two watches at once, even if it's a pendant/pin watch and bracelet watch.
- Be afraid to shop flea markets for jewelry bargains.
- Forget to clean your jewelry weekly.

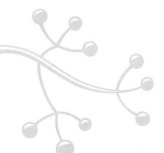

## Coco Chanel believed
that wearing too much real jewelry
was ostentatious.

# *Secrets of Scarves*

A scarf can double as a head wrap.

Use a scarf as a colorful belt.

Tie a large scarf around your waist
and it becomes a pareo.

A simple square scarf is a provocative face flatterer.

A scarf makes a wild necktie.

Fill in a suit with a scarf used as an ascot.

Tie a scarf on a purse to totally coordinate your outfit.

A small scarf makes a delightful wristband.

A rolled scarf is a necklace.

Any hat looks more festive with the addition of a scarf.

Purchase silk fabric and make your own scarf.

# Belts

## Chain Belts

Wear chain belts draped loosely around the hips.

## Colors

Wearing a belt in the same tone as a skirt or pant is more slimming.

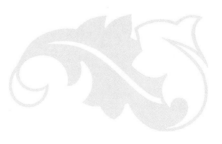

# Bargains

# Beauty on a Budget

It's easy to take charge of your beauty while maintaining your budget. It's a fun approach and easier than you think. Once you decide to devote just a little bit of extra time to read labels and explore new avenues, you will be amazed and gratified at just how much you can cut costs.

# Make it a Game

Finding that perfect bargain is a game you'll get hooked on. It's competitive. You're competing against other shoppers and you're competing against the merchandisers.

That's right; the stores will use every ploy to get you to make that purchase. They'll play relaxing music, scent the shopping area, and even use colors to invite you to pay more than you planned. Just like supermarkets, the item you're most likely to purchase will be conveniently located where you can reach and touch it.

## Ninety-Nine

Paying $24.99 seems to make us feel better than paying $25.00.

## The Coupon Game

Don't make that purchase just because you've brought a coupon along.

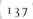

## Shampoos

There are very good brands available at excellent prices in drugstores. Enhance your shampoos with vodka (for shine) and vinegar (to remove residue). Rely on the conditioners you can easily make from scratch.

## Facials

Here's the facial that won't cost a cent and is highly beneficial. Steam your face by bending over a bowl of boiling water infused with your favorite herbal tea.

Fade dark circles under your eyes by placing the same cold tea bags over your eyes for about ten minutes.

## Haircuts

The best bargain for your hair is a good cut. If possible, pay extra for a top-of-the-line stylist (sometimes called a master stylist). More technically advanced haircuts will last longer (up to eight weeks, depending on the length). Save money by using chalk or powdered eye shadow to touch up telltale roots.

Cook two carrots until soft, then mash. Apply to your face, and let harden. Rinse with warm water. This vitamin A mask is beneficial and refreshing!

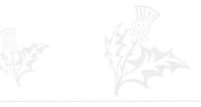

# Facial Toning

Tone up your facial muscles with water. Fill up your mouth with as much water as possible.

Hold it there for as long as you can. Allow the water pressure to do all the work for you.

Jut out your lower jaw. Gently raise your chin towards your nose, stretching your neck muscles. Then lower your chin back down to the starting position. Do this in the car, while talking on the phone, etc. This exercise will prevent "turkey jowl."

Open your eyes (as in a surprised expression) and try to reach your forehead. Do this several times.

# Home Treatments

Color and perfume your own Epsom salts for a delightful bath-time experience. Find salts in any drugstore. Store them in a big glass jar with a lid. Sprinkle in a few drops of food coloring, close the jar and shake it vigorously until the color is evenly distributed. Then pour it out onto a cookie sheet, and let it dry. You can speed things up by placing it in a warm oven for a half hour if you prefer. Perfume your salts with an essential oil or add a few drops of your favorite fragrance. Shake until there aren't any clumpy bits. You can add sea salts and baking soda to give it a different texture. Add a metal scoop, and you have your very own bath treatment.

While you're relaxing in the tub, increase the moisturizing effect by mashing two strawberries with two teaspoons of yogurt. Leave it on your face for 15 minutes. If you have any left over, rub it over the gum area to promote healthy gums.

To combat dryness, add a cup of oatmeal and a tablespoon of avocado oil to a warm bath. Soak for at least 15 minutes.

Remove excess oils from your face by mashing a tablespoon of pineapple and applying it to your face for 15 minutes before rinsing.

After shaving your legs, rub a slice of cucumber over them. Cleopatra used to have her legendary skin rubbed with cooked cucumber peels.

# Basic Bargain Tips

Don't buy an expensive cosmetic bag. A plastic pencil case is just the right size and transparent, to make finding things a snap. Some women prefer to use sealable sandwich bags for maximum space savings.

To extend the life of nail polish, clean the top of the bottle with a tissue after applying. Polish buildup allows air into the bottle, and the product will evaporate.

Almond oil will stop acrylic nails from dehydrating and coming away from the nail plate.

Save on accessories by shopping in girls' and teens' areas of department stores. You can save on such things as hair accessories, costume jewelry, purses, and scarves.

Get the most out of your fragrance by applying it only to pulse-point areas. A lot of perfume is wasted by spraying it into the air.

Save your broken lipstick, and pack it down in a small paint box or pill box. You now have a convenient lip gloss!

File the tips of your nails in one direction to make your manicure last longer.

Massage leftover hair conditioner into your cuticles.

Explore thrift and consignment shops when you aren't pressed for time. Since these types of shops don't have to worry much about cash flow, you'll find ten times the merchandise that you would find in a regular store. It may take patience and time, but the rewards are unending for the diligent bargain hunter.

Use oversized, outdated earrings to glamorize a pair of plain pumps or accessorize a jacket.

Add your own buttons to a pair of gloves for a designer look.

Add tassels to scarves for a rich style.

Cut buttons off old clothing, and recycle them for other clothes.

Witch hazel makes a great hair degreaser for dry shampooing.

Check to see if your insurance company will pay for sunscreen.

Use floor wax to protect shoes and handbags, and keep them shiny.

Have a clothing swap with friends, and see how great your shopping mistakes can look on someone else.

Use eye shadow as a liner by wetting it down and applying with a fine brush.

Mix your own colors by combining lipsticks and eye shadows.

Shop men's and boys' departments for great buys in sweaters, shirts, and workout clothing.

Use less of products than is recommended on the packaging. Many manufacturers tell you to use more so that you'll run out faster.

Use baby oil instead of makeup remover.

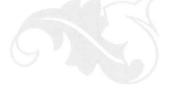
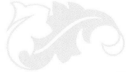

# Free Advice

Go to your local department store, and avail yourself of its personal shopping services. It won't cost you a dime, and you'll get the unbiased opinion that you can't get from friends, commissioned salespeople, or a "significant other." Don't bother to spend money on a professional image consultant. Every consultant I have ever interviewed uses rigid formulas for colors, matching fabrics, and other structured stuff that nobody has time for.

Plus, you'll hear a different opinion from each image consultant you meet. If you want several opinions, visit each of the major department stores in your area offering personal shopping services. Can't get out to a store? Many mail-order catalogs offer free phone advice. Be sure you have the company's catalog with you.

# It's Not a Bargain

If the buttons are poorly placed, it will gap.

If there's excess fabric, it will not be a flattering look.

Cheap lining. Fabrics like rayon will shrink once they're dry cleaned and will require alteration. The wrong lining can make the garment look dowdy.

Poor pocket placement should be avoided. When the pockets are too small, they can make the area that you're trying to disguise appear larger.

If the salesperson has to talk you into the purchase.

The maintenance makes the purchase ultimately too expensive. Check the label for cleaning recommendations before making your purchase.

If it pulls, bunches, rides up, or makes any kind of noise when you move in it.

## Best Time to Shop

You'll find that in most cases Friday night is the best time to shop. Stores usually start their sales on a Friday and very often stay open later.

## Shopping on eBay

eBay has become the ultimate marketplace for the perfect bargain. Almost everyone I know is buying or selling everything from their designer duds to Aunt Hilda's silverware. The eBay site makes it easy to make a purchase by simply registering a credit card.

Then you can browse or search, but like any auction don't let yourself get carried away. Make sure you thoroughly read the item description carefully, and look at the pictures the seller has included. If you have any questions about the item that aren't answered in the item's description, you can ask the seller about the item by clicking on the *Ask Seller a Question* link. Check the seller's feedback score and percentage of positive feedback right on the item page.

## Discount Stores

You can save a lot of money and avoid being hassled or ignored by shopping at drugstores and stores like Wal-Mart, Target, BJ's Wholesale, Costco, and other mixed merchandise and wholesale stores.

Use these stores to get the latest trends in cosmetics and colors.

Check the men's aisle for products like deodorant, shaving cream, disposable razors, and other non-gender items. They usually cost less. Try to find the unscented versions.

## No-Name Products

If you're afraid to try the store's own label, don't be. Many generic brands come from the same factory as the better-known product. Check the label and see if the ingredients are similar. They may not be in the same order, but if the active ingredient is the same you've got a winner.

## Grocery Store Finds

You can replicate expensive spa treatments with fresh produce and fruits. The bonus is that, although it may take a little longer to prepare, you're using the real product without the chemicals that do nothing for your face or body, but are only there to extend the shelf life.

# Bargain Weddings

How do you save on a wedding that runs anywhere from twenty to twenty-five thousand dollars and not appear cheesy?

Try to find a sample sale. Call local designers and ask when these sales will be held.

Find a seamstress you can trust. Ask around.

Consider a chain store. You'll find the fashions more affordable because synthetics and crystals are often used.

Ask the store if they will give you a discount if you purchase your entire bridal party's attire there.

Check out rental stores. Ask if alterations are allowed and if you are allowed to take the gown out in advance.

Make your own veil for a few dollars with a plastic comb, fabric, and embellishments from your local fabric store.

Look in your local department store's evening wear department.

Don't pay too much for your shoes. You'll probably only wear them once.

Don't feel that everything has to match, including the bridesmaid dresses.

*chapter* eleven

# Anti-Aging

# Simple Ways to Resist Aging

By cutting down or avoiding the following, you can help your skin to look younger a lot longer.

## The Sun

It's the number one reason why our skin ages. Wear sunscreen at all times, and don't forget protective clothing. Don't forget that the scalp also needs to be protected from the sun.

## Smoking

Early wrinkling occurs due to reduced levels of the oxygen needed to keep skin healthy. Smoking is the prime source of oxygen deprivation. Drinking lots of water will help counteract this.

## Alcohol

In excess, alcohol dehydrates the body and robs it of vitamins that keep skin both healthy and glowing. Never have an alcoholic drink without a chaser of ice water. It will detoxify the body and moderate the amount of alcohol intake.

## Improper Nutrition

The modern-day use of convenience foods encourages the formation of free radicals. These foods are high in processed fats and oils. Protection of the skin is possible by eating foods rich in vitamins A, C, and E. Fresh fruits and vegetables are particularly good for keeping the skin youthful. Supplementation may be necessary if you're not getting these nutrients in your foods.

## Stress

Stress causes the skin to become sensitive and prone to breakouts. Regular exercise and meditation will help diffuse its effects.

# Purchases Every Aging Beauty Must Make

## Three-Way Mirror

Especially after age forty, you must be certain you look as good going as you do coming. Unfortunately, some of the first signs of aging come from behind.

## Magnifying Mirror

There are things happening to your face and body, that the aging eye may not see. A five- to ten-times magnification mirror will help you to check on such exciting agers as age spots, facial hair, and wrinkles.

## Bronzing Powder

There is something to be said about the youthful look of a tan. Now you can do it safely. There is nothing short of plastic surgery that looks more rested. There's not one factor that will age you faster than the natural way of getting one. No, tanning beds are not any safer. Use bronzing powder liberally over the face, décolletage, and neck. It will take the years off quickly and efficiently and create a subtle reflection.

One of the most important ways to fight aging is with exercise. Even if you can't get into a total exercise program, you need to combine aerobic exercise with strength training to win the fight.

It's not necessary to join an expensive gym. You can get your heart pumping and increase your oxygen intake by taking the dog for a run, walking briskly to get your favorite coffee, gardening, or heavy housework. If you can sprint/run or jump rope, you will be building your muscles while building cardiovascular endurance. Your increased heart and lung performance will result in increased blood flow to the skin and resulting radiance.

## Strength Training

Strength training will give muscles more shape and keep skin tighter. It will also help relieve arthritic symptoms, increase bone density, improve posture, prevent lower back pain, and help raise metabolic rate. Free weights are inexpensive too. Start with five-pound weights and try to work up to ten-pound weights. You can even make your own with a two-liter bottle of soda filled with salt or sand.

# Plastic Surgery

Once considered extreme, cosmetic surgery is now being done on women and men of all incomes and ages. If you are considering plastic surgery, there are a few things that you need to know before searching out a plastic surgeon. If you've been looking in the mirror, pushing this, pulling that, and you're just tired of it, then you may feel that it's time. With all the new procedures available to you today, the most important thing is to be informed. Here are some available options.

## Eyes

In their thirties and forties, women will most likely choose an eye lift as their first procedure.

The eye lift of today is minimally invasive and no longer requires large incisions. Most surgeons agree that if a woman has excess eyelid skin, she is a good candidate. You can actually feel your brow and see if rests on or below the bone.

Anything below the bone would indicate a dropped brow.

## Endoscopic Brow Lift

An endoscope is used to raise the brow, anchoring it to the skull with tacks. It requires a shorter recovery time and is less traumatic than the traditional brow lift. A woman in her thirties or forties would be the best candidate for this type of surgery since her tissues are still firm enough for this approach. It is also used as a touch-up for eyes.

# Breast Surgery

Augmentation takes three to five weeks until swelling goes down and scars will almost always be visible.

Reduction is done to alleviate a variety of medical conditions including back pain, shoulder pain, headaches, and neck pain. Skin is taken from the bottom of the breast and the nipple and areola are relocated, but not detached. This procedure is almost always covered by insurance.

Lifts remove excess breast skin to raise and recontour sagging breasts. Scarring fades after two to three months and is usually done after significant weight loss.

# Tummy Tuck

This is the removal of excess stomach tissue often combined with liposuction and tightening of the muscle. It takes two to three months until a support garment is no longer needed.

A mini tummy tuck is a less invasive procedure that is used get rid of the middle to below-the-belt pouch, usually the result of pregnancies.

## Face

A full face-lift is most effective when done before the skin becomes thin. Healing time is about a month, but with the right cosmetics most women go out in about two weeks.

An endoscopic face-lift requires only four incisions, which include two inside the mouth and two behind the hairline, plus a few stitches to insure the tissue lift reestablishes high cheekbones and adds volume to the middle of the face. It can be used early or as a touch up after a full face-lift. It's out-patient surgery, but swelling and bruising can take up to a week to disappear.

## Don't Stop Changing

## Be Advised

Check out "Before" and "After" pictures of actual results.

Don't rely too much on computer imaging. Surgeons work on real people, not on machines.

Check to see that your surgeon is board certified at www.plasticsurgery.org.

Find a surgeon who will listen to your overall concerns.

Disregard anyone who does not completely explain the procedure and the risks involved.

Whatever you do, try not to become a caricature of your early years. Women who are guilty of this tend to wear the look that they had when they felt their most attractive. They don't look any younger. They look outdated. Our face and bodies change as we age and we need to adapt.

# Anti-Aging Rules to Live By

## Anti-Aging Rule #1

Update your makeup the way you update your wardrobe. The same applies to your hair color and style.

## Anti-Aging Rule #2

Increase your sleep. You know when you are getting enough rest when you wake up without an alarm clock. Sleep deprivation is the number one cause of premature aging (and the most frequently overlooked). Try to sleep in total darkness.

## Anti-Aging Rule #3

Eat and drink with a plan. Make every calorie work for your good health and beauty.

## Anti-Aging Rule #4

Lighten up! Don't obsess over every wrinkle and sag. You can fight aging but you can't eliminate it.

## Anti-Aging Rule #5

Age with grace and style and you'll always remain youthful.

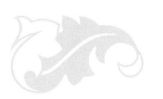

# chapter twelve

# Travel

# How to Pack

Packing is an art. You can be born with a gift for it. Do it enough, and you'll become an expert at it. It requires discipline, creativity, and a great deal of patience.

## Luggage

When you carry your luggage, you save time and hassles. The ideal travel wardrobe is like a well-planned itinerary. It will provide for everything that you need. Whether you need it for a week or a big weekend, you want to include just what you'll wear and nothing more. Always choose items that work with each other. Choose luggage that is both light and durable. Some luggage is heavy before anything is packed in it. This is the last luggage you would ever want to carry. Modern materials are now available that weigh next to nothing and perform the job beautifully and durably. Also avoid luggage that has no bend or give to it.

## Colors

This area requires a good deal of restraint, but try to stick to two colors when packing. For instance, black and ivory are two colors that work well when traveling. You'll add one more color for dimension and accent. If you're choosing black and ivory, add a little red for a dash of pizzazz.

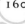

## Clothes

Take those few key pieces (trousers, shorts, skirt, jacket) according to the climate you are visiting, and let your accessories carry you through. Lay everything out on the bed, and create different combinations before packing.

## Packing

Bulky or heavy items should be placed at the very bottom and sides of the suitcase. This prevents them from falling down and wrinkling clothing as soon as the suitcase is picked up. Fill shoes with socks and underwear, and slip them into plastic bags to protect your clothing. Place high heels with the heel toward the middle, so that they won't ruin your luggage. Plastic bags are slippery, so you can pack a lot more. Perfume bottles should be placed inside shoes. Not only will that protect the bottle, but it also maintains the shape of the shoe. Roll whatever you can and keep it tight and small with a rubber band.

## Cosmetics

Try to find a compact beauty case. If you like to hang your cosmetics from the back of the bathroom door hook, choose a roll-type cosmetics bag. Fill your cosmetics bag with travel-sized items. You should be able to go to your local department store, and get sample sizes of just about every cosmetic you will need. Seal all toiletries in a plastic bag.

## Jewelry

When packing jewelry, there are tricks that every smart traveler uses. If you're planning to bring some necklaces along, run them through a straw and clasp. This prevents knots and tangles.

# Packing Tricks

Fold long, easily wrinkled fabrics around sturdier ones. For instance, pack your elegant silk blouse around your jeans.

Don't pack anything you don't wear at home.

Pack a scarf or two. You'll find this is one of the most useful travel items. You can wear it as a sarong, use it as a swimsuit cover, use it in place of a blouse to wear under suits, and even use it to strategically cover stains.

Upon arrival at your hotel, unpack everything and hang any wrinkled garments in the shower to steam away wrinkling. Always include a sewing kit, scissors, and a clothes brush or tape.

A hairdryer takes on another life when traveling. It's a quick dryer for hose, lingerie, and small stains. Most hotels have them, but call ahead to confirm.

The plastic bags you've used in packing will be used at your destination for laundry and wet swimsuit storage.

Use a good-sized tote to carry on anything you consider a necessity. That usually includes eyeglasses or contact lens items, money, camera, medications, real jewelry, passport, and reading materials.

Pack a foldaway bag for the souvenirs you won't be able to live without.

Bring a small address book or personal organizer for addresses and emergency phone numbers.

When traveling abroad, always take a skirt.

# In the Air

Drink plenty of water to counteract the drying effects of "canned" air.

Wear glasses instead of contact lenses.

Grab a pillow and blanket upon boarding.

Bring a toothbrush and toothpaste for long flights.

Always wear comfortable clothing.

Don't drink more than one alcoholic beverage. It's very dehydrating.

Bring slippers or slipper socks to keep your feet warm when you slip off your shoes.

Dress in layers so you can add or subtract as the temperature in the cabin changes.

# Did You Know?

Your shoes may not fit at the end of your flight. Your feet will swell considerably in the air, so be sure that your shoes are a bit roomy starting out. Mules or skids are the best traveling shoes.

Your hair will become full of static during your flight. That's because of the dry air. Use a silicone-based de-frizzer to coat it.

Epsom salts will relieve jet lag. After a flight, add 3 cups of Epsom salts to your bath water. The magnesium chloride will draw out wastes and leave you feeling tranquil.

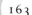

## Special Destinations

### Cold Weather Vacations

Always wear a moisturizing sunscreen of at least 30 SPF.

Use powder-based foundation so that there will be no rub-off on your scarf.

To keep color on your lips, line the entire lip with pencil and finish off with a lip balm.

Don't bother with blush. The outdoors will give you a natural glow.

A ponytail or braids will control long hair, and is perfectly acceptable on the slopes or trails.
Avoid hat head by wearing earmuffs or a headband.

Use extra conditioning treatments on your hair to avoid static from hats

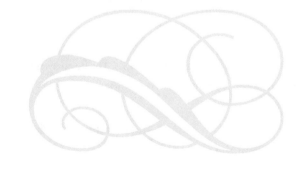

## Hot Weather Vacations

Good sunglasses are essential for eye safety and protection against wrinkles. Check for UV protection before you buy.

Wear clothes with a built-in UV block. Pure silk, high-shine polyester, and terry cloth are sun blockers. Stay away from bleached cottons and crepes.

Stage your workout in the pool. The natural buoyancy causes the muscles to work harder, and it feels just great.

Use the beach's sand to exfoliate your skin. Rub it all over those rough spots.

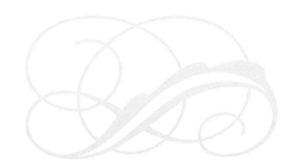

Leave your hair conditioner on while in the sun. It acts like a heat cap.

Sprinkle talcum powder into shoes before wearing.

Wear cotton underclothing.

Stay cool with loose-fitting clothing and waistbands.

# *Maintaining and Organizing*

# *Beauty*

# Protect Your Investments

After spending a small fortune on your wardrobe, shoes, and accessories, it just doesn't make any sense not to keep your things in good repair. You take care of your car, your kids, and your home. Why won't you give yourself the same consideration? It doesn't take that long, and it's well worth the effort. It's guaranteed to make life easier for you in the long run.

# The Big Cleanup

Here's how to make your wardrobe more wearable.

1. Go through your closet and get rid of anything you haven't worn in two seasons.
2. Get rid of mistakes. If it doesn't have any place to go, give it one—your local charity or eBay!
3. Toss out what doesn't fit. Face reality. It hurts more to look at that piece of clothing than it does to clear it out. Your closet should be totally ready to go.
4. Make repairs. Chances are, the garment is not being utilized because it's simply not ready.
5. Items you are absolutely forever attached to must be stored.
6. Hang clothes by category, outfit, or possibilities.
7. Final Rule: Throw away anything you don't want, use, or love.

# Clothes Care

Check dry cleaning instructions. Throwing a delicate fabric into the washing machine will ruin its finish.

⁂

Invest in padded hangers. Wire hangers can leave shoulder marks or ridges.

⁂

Wrap hangers in tissue paper to support heavier clothing.

⁂

Keep leather and suede garments and shoes supple by treating them with a protective cream.

⁂

Iron inside out to avoid dulling the gleam of the fabric.

⁂

Remove lint from knits and woolens by shaving the surface with an electric razor or sweater shaver.

⁂

Treat shoes and bags with a stain repellent.

Wash or dry clean clothing before storing. Moths are less attracted to clean clothes.

⁂

Dry cleaning is the quickest way to freshen a tired garment.

⁂

When storing clothes, keep moths away by putting some dry bay leaves between layers in storage boxes and garment bags. Bay leaves won't leave the distasteful odor found in mothballs.

⁂

Jackets must be hung to keep their shape. Stuff arms with tissue paper or newspaper.

⁂

Always button and zip clothing to hang properly and to maintain space in your closet.

⁂

Fold sweaters. Hanging them will cause them to mysteriously grow!

Apply a thin coat of clear nail polish or nail hardener to pearl buttons to restore their luster and make them more durable.

To remove deodorant stains, rub clothing with a little ammonia before laundering. For regular stains, mix three parts baking soda to two parts vinegar.

Instead of buying expensive garment bags to protect your hanging clothes from fading, cover them with old pillowcases.

Perfume padded hangers to scent your clothing.

Altering clothing gives it a new life. Long skirts can be shortened, wide pants can be taken in, and shoulder pads can be easily removed.

# Shoes

Use an old-fashioned rubber eraser to remove grime from suede and fabric shoes.

Use a soft cloth or brush (not wire) to loosen surface dirt.

A black felt-tip pen can color in scuff marks.

Store your boots on boot trees. If you don't have room, stuff them as much as possible with newspaper.

Pull out the inner sole of your shoe or boot and let it air out periodically.

Never let shoes dry near a radiator or heating duct. Too much heat may crack the leather and shrink the skin.

Go easy on waterproofing and harsh chemical treatments. Some of the ones on the market today can do as much harm as good. Floor wax is a safe and inexpensive weatherproofer.

To remove salt stains from boots, dampen a sponge with white vinegar. Gently blot away marks.

To rid suede of water marks, brush against the grain. Allow it to dry. If it's a soft suede, fill with tissue or newspaper to ensure the integrity of the shape.

Erase dark marks from pale leather by dabbing with nail polish remover.

Blot grease stains with a paper towel. Follow up by massaging with talcum powder for five minutes. Brush away with a soft brush.

Clean patent leather with a glass cleaner. Of course, the traditional "spit" routine always works too.

# Accessories

When cleaning a handbag, remove the contents and stuff it with newspapers or plastic.

For leather or suede gloves, stuff the fingers with paper towels or toilet paper tubes. Place the gloves on top of a soda bottle to dry.

Brush your jewelry with baking soda or toothpaste.

Use only the mildest soap when cleaning pearls.

Get your eyeglasses to stay put by dabbing clear nail polish on top of the screws.

# Organization

Take your earrings and fasten them through the holes of a button. This will keep them from getting separated.

Gather up all your pins and brooches. Decorate them on a cork bulletin board. They will be in sight and available. No more rummaging in drawers for those jewels.

Use old stuffed pillows to create pin art. If you are a pin collector, use a pillow for each color theme, and you will have created a colorful display. After all, isn't jewelry art?

Use a hanger to display all your necklaces. This will eliminate the unnecessary tangling and knotting created by throwing long chains into jewelry boxes.

## Improvise!

If you don't have enough compartments in your purse, attach Velcro to your keys and compact and attach it to the lining.

Dealing with a small closet? Hooks are great space savers. Use them for everything from bathrobes to handbags.

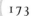

# Miscellaneous

Use the shampoos and conditioners you've never liked to wash your hair and makeup brushes. Shampoo and soak everything! Rinse with conditioner. They will be in soft, silky shape and will make your cosmetics and hair flow beautifully!

If you can smell any of your cosmetics, then throw them away immediately. If you're on a budget, always look for oil-free cosmetics. They last a lot longer.

Eye makeup has the shortest shelf life. Because eyes are so easily irritated, eye makeup contains less preservatives. Keeping any eyeliner or mascara more than six months is putting you at risk for eye infections.

It's not necessarily a good deal to purchase larger containers. Bacteria builds up if a product is not used right away.

# Facts about Fragrances

Perfumes don't last forever. Once you open a bottle, use it until it's empty. Limit your perfume's exposure to the air. Fragrance is very much like wine; once it's open, it starts to disintegrate. Women who line their boudoirs with bottles of various fragrances will unfortunately find that eventually, the quality will be jeopardized. Eventually, some of them will sour. Once a perfume or cologne starts to smell like alcohol or vinegar, it's time to toss it.

Foods affect natural body odors and the fragrance of perfumes. That's why one scent will smell one way on a vegetarian, and another on a meat eater. Fragrances will smell differently on people who eat garlicky foods as opposed to those who eat more bland foods. Fragrance is also different at certain times of a woman's menstrual cycle. Other factors affecting your perfume's fragrance are vitamins, cigarettes, and certain drugs.

Every night, plan to bathe in your favorite fragrance, and mend your mind from the day's stresses. Your bathroom is one room in your home that is made for sensory pleasures. Add a little mood music, and you've created your own aromatherapy experience. Don't forget the candles.

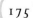

# *Intimate*
# *Beauty*

## Home Sweet Spa

Every woman deserves an area in her home that is entirely hers. If you do not have that space, begin to create one. It will be your own laboratory, where you can establish a home "spa." This area will be the one place you will use to store your own ideas and creations, and try some of the tips that I will share with you in this chapter.

# Make Your Own Toothpaste

In my work, I have come into contact with some inventive beauties and some real space cadets. Would you believe that there are some models using bathroom cleansers in an effort to whiten their teeth? These young beauties (who won't be lovely for long) are under the false impression that they can whiten their teeth with Comet and Ajax. Not only will this practice wear the enamel away, but it is also dangerous!

There are secret recipes being passed around that *will* safely whiten your teeth, will not cost you an arm and a leg, and will not cause you to lose your enamel.

## Hydrogen Peroxide

Mix 1 teaspoon of hydrogen peroxide and 1 teaspoon of baking soda. Brush your teeth with this mixture once a week. Be very careful not to swallow! This formula will reduce tartar and remove coffee and tea stains.

Dip unwaxed dental floss in hydrogen peroxide to brighten spaces between teeth where discoloration often starts.

## Burned Toast

It may sound strange, but burned toast is effective in whitening teeth. Pound a couple of slices into a powder and add a few drops of peppermint oil. The charcoal in the toast is the key ingredient.

## Salt

Mix 3 tablespoons of baking soda with 2 tablespoons of salt for a safe and natural cleanser for teeth.

## fourteen

## Do-It-Yourself Mouthwashes

### Tea Wash

Boil a strong cup of mint (peppermint, spearmint, etc.) tea. Cool and rinse.

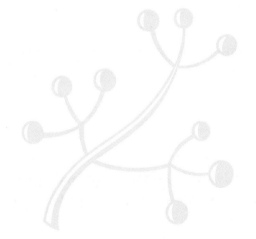

### Honey/Clove Rinse

Mix 1/4 cup of honey with 1 teaspoon of ground cloves. This mouthwash can be thinned down if desired.

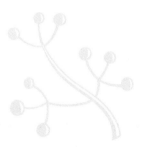

# Agony of the Feet

When purchasing a heel higher than one inch, go up a half size. There's some natural swelling that occurs that necessitates advancing at least half a size in order to accommodate the toe area. This is one time when smaller is not more attractive. A tight shoe bulges the foot out, not to mention what it does for the wearer's expression. A larger shoe actually gives the foot a longer, more graceful line.

## Change Shoes

Try not to wear the same pair of shoes two days in a row. Give them at least 24 hours to air out.

## Use an Antiperspirant

The foot contains more sweat glands than the underarm area. Don't waste that precious money on expensive foot powders and other foot remedies. Not only is this cosmetically important, but it is key in keeping bacteria at bay.

## Soak Your Feet

At least once a week, steep 4 tea bags (purchase an inexpensive brand because it will contain a larger content of tannic acid) in 2 cups of boiling water for at least 5 minutes. Add 2 cups of cool water. Soak for up to 30 minutes. Note: Don't use herbal tea because it's the tannic acid that will cause proteins in the skin to bond. This thickens the skin and blocks many of its sweat pores.

# The Healthy Breast

## Wear a Bra

The chest muscles don't provide enough support to go braless, no matter how small your breasts are.

Keep your weight constant. Yo-yo dieting can cause the breasts to sag.

When trying on a bra, lean way over to make sure breasts fit snugly and comfortably in cups.

## Exercise in the Proper Bra

If your breasts feel tender after a workout, you're probably not wearing a bra that is supportive enough.

A sports bra should be made of material that prevents sweat from gathering underneath and between the breasts.

Make sure that the straps don't slip while running or jumping.

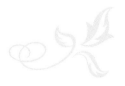

## Perspiration

Perspiration can collect in the cleavage and especially under the bust. Keep the area dry by dusting the breasts with talcum powder before dressing.

## Bulges

Should you find yourself "pouring out" of your bra, choose a style with more support at the sides and underneath.

## Bathing

The beauty benefits of bathing are many. Use this time as a restorative, a spa, and personal time.

## Temperature

Keep water warm, rather than hot. A too-hot bath strips the skin of moisture and will leave you feeling dehydrated.

## Additives

### TEA

Tie a tea bag under the faucet so that the water will run through the bag. Use your favorite herbal teas, which will scent the water and you. The aroma will relax and invigorate you.

### ALKA-SELTZER

Toss a tablet into your tub and your bath will fill up with tiny bubbles, skin softeners, and other good things.

### BABY OIL

Soften water and your skin to silken elegance with a splash of baby oil.

# Intimate Information

## Hair Removal

Getting rid of hair is so much fun, isn't it? Here are some pointers that I hope will make the job a bit less tedious.

Don't shave right after getting out of bed. Skin tends to be puffy in the morning, and stubble is not as visible. Try to wait a half hour if you can.

Make sure hair is well-moistened. Use shaving cream, soap, or other softener.

Start at ankles, go to bikini line, and then to under-arms. This gives coarser hair a chance to soften.

Avoid getting waxed just before or during your period. You are more sensitive to pain at this time.

Tweeze hair in the tub. It's easier to tweeze when skin's warm and soft.

Shave opposite hair growth. It prevents hairs from curling under the skin and becoming ingrown.

Numb areas with witch hazel or ice to lessen pain.

### THE BIKINI AREA

The bikini line can be difficult to shave because the hair grows in so many different directions. Always prepare the skin with soap and water. Don't stop shaving the bikini area just because the colder months have set in and you've stopped wearing a bathing suit. Discontinuing to shave this area will cause it to become overly sensitive. So when the warmer months return, you'll literally have to "break in" that area again. Ouch!

Some women choose to shave or trim their pubic hair for hygienic purposes as well as appearance. Use caution when doing so. Use small scissors for safety.

Don't shave your bikini line before going to the beach if you're skin is prone to irritation. You risk a rash or mottled skin.

## UNDERARMS

Hair also grows in different directions in the underarm area. Teach yourself to shave up and down and sideways. Always prep this area thoroughly.

## LOOFAH YOUR LEGS

Try to give your legs a light scrub with a loofah before you shave them. This will get rid of all the excess dead skin cells that may otherwise clog up your razor. If you use a double-edge razor, then switch to a single-edge one.

# Deodorants

There are more deodorants on the market than ever. The skinny on deodorants is that there's a lot of hype in the marketing. Sweat is sweat, whether it's on a man or woman. Models don't want to lose big jobs by ruining a designer dress with perspiration. You won't find any fancy, delicate flowery deodorants in a model's bag. Go get the strongest (yes, the ones made for a man) antiperspirant that you can find, and forget about the fancy, overpriced, weak stuff.

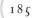

## Bloat

If you have a tendency toward excess bloating, don't chew gum, sip through a straw, or drink from a bottle. These cause you to swallow air, which goes to your stomach.

## Baring Skin

Make sure to wash after shampooing and conditioning your hair. Hair products leave a residue of oil on your shoulders and back.

Always wear sunscreen on exposed chest and back areas.

## Cellulite

The methods of getting rid of cellulite are controversial to say the least. The cottage cheese that seems to gather on the back of the thighs and other spots are best eliminated by working it off in an aerobic program. Spot exercises fail miserably. Running, walking, dancing, swimming, and skating rev up the body's metabolism for burning fat throughout the body.

Work off cellulite in your tub. Lie on your stomach, bend one knee, raise and lower heel to the ceiling. Try not to drown doing this exercise.

Some cellulite marks that are unsightly can be diminished with massage. Break open a vitamin E capsule with a safety pin (1,000 units) and rub into those pesky areas.

# Sleep for Beauty

There can be no doubt about it. When we don't get enough sleep, we don't look well. Most of us need at least eight hours of uninterrupted sleep. Tossing and turning or awakening several times a night is detrimental not only to your looks, but to your overall psyche. Unfortunately, it's not always so easy to fall asleep and stay asleep. But there are ways to put the odds in your favor.

## Melatonin

This is the supplement you've been reading about, "nature's sleeping pill." Taken twenty minutes before bedtime, melatonin is certainly worth a try. Some users have expressed concern about nightmarish dreams, while others have praised the vivid, lucid dreams they have been experiencing. Although still controversial, this supplement has also been linked to anti-aging properties.

## Eat Early

There are very important reasons not to eat past 5 or 6 p.m. Late-night eating makes for difficulty in sleeping. You will end up wide awake, while your body is trying to digest your last meal. If you've eaten certain kinds of foods, you'll experience painful heartburn. Plus, as every successful dieter knows, those late meals are not good for weight reduction.

## Scent Your Pillow

Add a few drops of eucalyptus (available at health stores and natural supermarkets) to promote breathing. Stuffy nasal passages, whether due to a cold, flu, or allergies, can cause you to awaken during the night. Scientists have discovered that when you have a cold, you awaken up to a hundred times, although you may not be aware of it.

## Drink Tea

Several teas on the market today have been found to be helpful in inducing sleep. Although chamomile tea promotes sleep, it's also a diuretic, defeating its purpose.

## Set Your Clock

Try to go to sleep and wake up at the same time every day, including weekends. Your body will try to adjust to a regular schedule. Sleeping in on weekends will disrupt your body's inner clock.

## Sleeping on Your Back

Here's an age-old beauty secret that you won't pay a cent for, but could save you dozens of wrinkles over the years. Wrinkles form on the side you sleep on. If you can't train yourself to remain on your back, invest in a satin pillow. Your face is going to slide around all night on this pillowcase, discouraging the wrinkling effect.

## Keep It Cool

In an offbeat way, a slightly cool room is in fact, a beauty treatment. A room that is too hot can cause you to perspire. This increases oil production, which clogs the skin's pores. Equally important is to sleep on (and in) bed clothing that "breathes."

## Get Plenty of Exercise

Although going through a rigorous workout routine just before bed can keep you awake, regular exercise may help you to sleep longer and more soundly. If you should find yourself "wired," do some easy stretching to relax and soothe your muscles and promote those zzzz's.

## Wash Off Your Makeup

*Please* remove every bit of face and eye makeup before getting into bed. Failing to do so can cause bacteria buildup and acne.

## Take a Bath

A warm bath will relax the body into a "ready for sleep" mode. Use bathing as a prelude to a night of beautiful dreams.

## Get Gorgeous

Use the heaviest moisturizer you can find to make up for the loss of water during the night.

Fight free radicals during the night by puncturing a vitamin C capsule and adding it to your night cream. Elevate your head with a firm pillow to eliminate puffiness.

# Tips for the Home

Stop paying for a housekeeper. Blast that stereo, then clean and exercise at the same time.

Choose underwear that matches your skin tone. Don't try to match your clothing.

Keep an aloe vera plant in your house. Break it open and use it to heal a sunburn. Apply it to your face as a refresher.

Grow parsley for fresh breath.

Keep cucumbers for emergency eye compresses.

Stock up on baking soda. Use it to soothe your skin in the bath. Brush your teeth with it. Clean your jewelry.

Rely on lemons to remove stains on teeth, soften hard skin on elbows and knees, and rinse your hair.

# chapter fifteen

# Supplementing Beauty

## That Extra Edge

Whether you're looking to accelerate weight loss, show skin improvement, or enhance overall health, there are vitamins and supplements available to help. You'll find expensive combination formulas that you can purchase, and many name brands that you are familiar with and trust, but if you are armed with accurate information you can make up your own combinations and get more powerful ingredients at a much lower cost. You'll also have the ability to purchase more generic brands because you will know exactly what you're getting in the product.

## Supplements for Weight Loss

### Garcinia Cambogia

Garcinia cambogia is a yellow fruit from Southeast Asia. Used in cooking, the garcinia extract is added to make meals more filling. Said to aid digestion, it contains hydroxyl citric acid, which is similar to the citric acid found in citrus fruits.

Available in pill form and in bars at health food stores, garcinia cambogia has taken the natural weight loss industry by storm. It helps control the appetite.

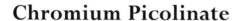

## Chromium Picolinate

Scientists have discovered that people who lack chromium in their bodies carry extra weight. The supplement chromium picolinate and chromium polynicotate have been around for a few years. It is an essential dietary nutrient that plays an important role in processing fat and carbohydrates. Many users report that it cuts sweet cravings, too. You could use this supplement if your diet is lacking chromium-rich foods. These foods include mushrooms, apples, broccoli, and cheese. The recommended daily allowance is anywhere from 200 to 400 micrograms. Supplements are usually sold in 200 micrograms or mixed with other products in varying amounts. This product is readily available in drugstores, health food stores, supermarkets, and general merchandisers.

## L-Carnitine

This supplement is reported to accelerate the benefits of chromium. Leading fitness buffs and die-hard weight watchers take the two together. It is sold as a separate unit and in combination with other supplements. L-Carnitine is an amino acid that is alleged to be in short supply in many diets. The recommended dosage for this supplement is from 500 to 1000 mg daily.

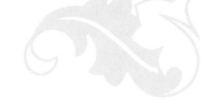

## Supplements for Youth

### DHEA

This supplement is short for dehydroepiandrosterone, a hormone made by the adrenal glands, located just above the kidneys. Being touted as the "fountain of youth," benefits reported include more energy (including sexual energy), and better skin and hair. Formerly only available by prescription, DHEA is now sold at drugstores and health food stores. Recommended dosage is from 25 to 50 mg.

### Vinegar

Ancient healers have used vinegar for thousands of years. Take two teaspoonfuls of vinegar mixed with a glass of water at each meal. The vinegar will help your body to burn fat, rather than store it. Use any vinegar that appeals to you. Apple cider vinegar is a delicious flavor to try. Vinegar is a natural storehouse of vitamins and minerals.

# Supplements for a More Beautiful Life

Our attitudes have really changed toward supplements. I don't know of a beauty today who does not take her daily supply of vitamins and minerals in capsule form. For looks, vitality, and general well-being, we would have to consume too many calories if we were to rely on food during the day. That's why supplements are now playing such an important role in the regimens of the world's most beautiful women. In addition to their multivitamins, here are the supplements most often mentioned.

## Vitamin A

Take this supplement to regulate skin hydration, aid eyesight, and repair skin and nails.

## Vitamin B

This important vitamin keeps skin smooth, promotes hair and nail growth, and improves circulation.

## Vitamin C

Available in several forms, it is quickly becoming the darling of the cosmetics industry. Vitamin C prolongs the life of vitamin E, and protects immune cells in the skin to fight off cancer and other sun-related diseases. It also has been proven to fade age spots and other pigment irregularities. Vitamin C fends off colds, and regenerates the skin.

## Vitamin E

Known as the skin vitamin, it has properties to heal scar tissue, fight damage, and neutralize damaging free radicals that come from UV rays.

## Ginkgo Biloba

Good circulation is vital to a healthy brain to supply it with the food and oxygen it needs. Ginkgo, derived from the oldest living tree, has many benefits. It increases alertness, improves memory, and lowers cholesterol levels. But more important (to our looks), there's evidence that ginkgo may be the most potent anti-ager ever! The only problem I have come across is that there's no agreed-upon standard for the right amount to take. About 40 mg seems to be the recommended dosage from most sources I have solicited.

## Beta Carotene

This vitamin A precursor protects cell membrane and skin cells from free radical attack. In everyday language, beta carotene makes the skin stay moist, supple, and youthful.

## Pycnogenol

A compound from the French maritime pine, this is a most powerful antioxidant that acts in a similar way as vitamin E, but with fifty times the strength. It boasts twenty times the strength of vitamin C. Use it to protect cell membranes from sun damage.

## Echinacea

Rich in polysaccharides, echinacea helps to activate the immune cells. It also naturally inhibits inflammation. Widely used in Europe, take it only when you feel an illness coming on. It has no cumulative effects.

## Grape Seeds

Antioxidants in grape seeds protect the thin walls of blood vessels from losing their strength. Beauties use it to prevent and correct the appearance of spider veins.

## Licorice Root

Long used in Germany, this helps with vitamin absorption and the prevention of ulcers.

## Seaweed

What you used to avoid at the beach has many health benefits. It's sold in both dried form and in tablets. You can reconstitute it and add it to your salads and soups as many models do. If seaweed doesn't exactly tempt your taste buds, go for the tablets. The most popular tablets are Dulse and Kelp. Take it for its rehydrating benefits. Seaweed can also boost a sluggish thyroid.

## Evening Primrose Oil

Particularly popular in England, it benefits the skin and hair, and is said to aid in hair restoration.

## Garlic

Take the deodorized version in tablet form to lower high blood pressure and cholesterol.

## Lavender Oil

Use it in drop form in the bath to alleviate stress, and ease headache pain.

## Ginger

It prevents motion sickness and relieves nausea. Ginger is also reported to prevent and heal ulcers.

## Grapefruit Seed Extract

Made from the seeds and pulp of grapefruits, grapefruit seed extract is receiving praise from both holistic and mainstream medical researchers. Its properties boost the immune system and are proclaimed to be an alternative to antibiotics. It is reported to fight bacteria, viruses, and parasites, which is why it is most often used for flus, colds, sore throats, and even yeast infections.

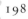

## Cat's Claw

Known as the Peruvian wonder herb, cat's claw comes out of the ancient rainforest of the Amazon. A natural antioxidant, one of the major benefits is that it is anti-edemic (it takes down swelling). Use it for swollen ankles, bloating, and PMS.

## Bee Pollen

The buzz on bee pollen is that it gives you an extra energy lift. Be sure to take small doses of it in the beginning. Some users have found that they are allergic to it. It's used as an alternative to coffee by holistic practitioners.

## Ginseng

This popular supplement has many health and longevity benefits. It improves energy levels and enhances mental alertness. It has immune strengthening benefits and can lower cholesterol levels. Ginseng is reported to decrease the chance of heart disease, and to increase good (HDL) cholesterol levels.

## Selenium

Take this vitamin to enhance the effects of vitamin E. Selenium has a close metabolic interrelationship with vitamin E and aids in body growth.

## Royal Jelly

Here is one of the most enduringly popular food supplements. Swathed in the mysteries of ancient China and the East where it was first discovered,

Royal jelly, in its raw state, is a unique, high-protein food. It's produced by bees and fed to their offspring. Used as a food supplement, it is available in both capsule and liquid forms. Loyal followers prefer the liquid because it can be more easily absorbed into the system. Also use it to boost your energy levels.

# Wheat Grass Juice

Here's yet another purported natural energy enhancer. It is also used in homeopathic healing of some diseases and is a staple of raw food diets.

# Spirulina

Used by weight-conscious beauties worldwide, spirulina is believed to suppress the appetite. It's widely available in drugstores and is inexpensive.

# Silica

Many people swear by silica for radiant skin, luxurious hair, and rapid, strong nail growth. It also provides collagen to the body. It is available in tablets and is also known as a hair, skin, and nail vitamin.

# Coenzyme Q-10

Produced in the body naturally, it is being hailed as a powerful weapon against heart disease. Research also suggests that it may prolong youth and enhance the power of the brain. Mice given coenzyme Q-10 remained extremely active into old age and tended to live longer. The results did not come in until the rats grew old, which makes Q-10 more of an insurance policy than an overnight miracle. The recommended dosage is 75 mg to 150 mg.

## Valerian Root

For those who can't take melatonin, valerian root is a mild tranquilizer and sleep aid.

## Cranberry

Taken as a powdered concentrate, cranberry prevents recurrence of urinary tract infections.

## The Best Time to Take Supplements

Although the specific hour is not really important, what is necessary is that you take your supplements at the same time each day. Make them part of your routine. Some supplements are better absorbed with food. Follow the directions found on each label.

# chapter sixteen

# Beauty Emergencies

## *Don't Panic*

When you have a beauty emergency, don't panic! You have items in your home or medicine cabinet that you will get you through almost any kind of beauty catastrophe.

In this chapter I'm happy to share these "in a pinch" beauty secrets. They are coveted by celebrities, makeup artists, and models, and they really work. They've been around for years because sometimes no matter what, "life happens."

# Skin Emergencies

## Emerging Pimple

To stop redness and swelling in an emergency situation (job interview, reunion, wedding), ask your doctor for a cortisone injection. It calms down a pimple almost instantly. If you can't get to your dermatologist, you can reduce redness and swelling by dabbing on a drop of drugstore cortisone cream, hemorrhoid cream, or eye drops.

### OVERNIGHT TREATMENT
Rub ice on an emerging pimple for 30 to 40 seconds. Apply clove oil and leave it on until it dries completely.

### TEA TREE OIL
Massage a touch of tee tree oil around the area of the pimple to anesthetize it and encourage healing. Use a nonliquid concealer to match your foundation.

Dab a little on the blemish, wait a couple of seconds, then blend lightly with a fingertip. Dust with loose powder.

## Acne Rash

Take yellow eye shadow and mix it with your concealer. Apply it to the area and allow to dry. Then cover with your regular foundation. Even it out by gently blotting your face with a separated tissue.

## Puffy Eyes

Take some cold spoons and place them under the eye area. Simply run them under cold water for a few seconds, or even better, keep them in the freezer so they'll be ready when it's the "morning after" or when you just didn't get enough sleep.

## Body Chafing

If there's no medicated powder around, use a little cornstarch. It contains fabulous absorbing powers, and you may find it even more effective.

## Chapped Lips

Rub on a little petroleum jelly, then use a toothbrush to brush your lips in little circular motions. The toothbrush will exfoliate the dead skin while the petroleum jelly will provide a base so your lipstick glides on.

## Cold Sore

There are medications for cold sores and fever blisters. If you don't have any on hand, take an aspirin and apply it, slightly dampened, to the sore. Hold it there for at least three minutes.

Keep the sore and its surrounding area clean and dry to fight bacteria.

Eat a bland diet, avoiding chocolate, nuts, or gelatin-based products. These foods may irritate the sore and cause further infection.

## Excess Self-Tanner

Soak in a warm bath for about 20 minutes using baking soda as body scrub.

## Bad Sunburn

Take an aspirin to reduce the inflammation. Bathe in a tub of vinegar and warm water (use about a pint of vinegar). Moisturize the skin with yogurt or nonfat milk.

## Fragrance Overload

Swab the skin with an alcohol-soaked cotton pad. Then smooth on unscented lotion to remoisturize and help diffuse the fragrance even further.

# Makeup Emergencies

## Eyeliner Won't Stay On

For eyeliner that goes on darker and stays on longer, eye drops will do the trick.

Add a little eye redness reliever to cake liner or powdered eye shadow and then apply along the lid with an angled brush. You get a perfectly smooth line that will last all night.

## Big Under-Eye Circles

Apply a concealer at least a half-shade lighter than your skin tone. Use it after applying your foundation. Mix a bit of blue eye shadow with moisturizer. Follow with foundation.

## No Makeup Remover

If you've run out of makeup remover, use olive oil. In the beauty industry, extra-virgin olive oil is preferred. It doesn't clog pores or cause breakouts.

## Clumped Mascara

Dip a cotton swab in makeup remover and then squeeze until it's almost dry. Go over lashes with the swab to remove any excess. A folded tissue placed under lower lashes will catch anything. Comb lashes while they're damp, and then blink against a tissue to blot excess as well as guard against smudges.

## Over-Blushed

If instead of getting a rosy glow you ended up looking like a clown, then simply take a big fluffy powder puff and press it onto your cheeks to lift excess color away. Take another clean puff, and apply a layer of loose powder on top.

## Day-to-Evening Makeup in Minutes

Go deeper with your lips. First, line your lip with a lip liner, matching your lipstick, and apply lipstick. Finish with a neutral pencil to fill the outer rim of the lips.

To make eyelashes appear longer, apply a coat of mascara and then use a cotton swab to dust the lashes with loose powder; add a second coat of mascara.

Create a smoky eye with petroleum jelly. Line the top and bottom lash lines with a dark pencil. Put a thin layer of petroleum jelly over the lid and blink, and you'll have the desired smudged look.

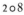

# Hair Emergencies

## Hair Product Greasies

A handful of oatmeal will absorb excess grease and product. Just rub the flakes into your hair and brush them out onto a newspaper. To get your volume back, bend over at your waist and apply a light mist of hair spray. Then add lift at the roots by lifting your hair in sections and blow-drying using your fingers.

## Hair Color Gone Green

Green-tinted hair, most obvious on blondes, is caused by substances such as nickel and chlorine that are found in swimming pools and in hard and well water. You can get rid of this color by using 5 aspirin dissolved in 1/3 cup of shampoo. Shampoo thoroughly, and then condition well.

## Visible Hair Roots

When you have hair growth that is truly noticeable, always improvise with something that you can eventually wash out. My favorite is to take powdered eye shadow matching the color as close to the hair color as possible, and work it with my finger into the growth. Of course, yellow is perfect for blondes, and there are lots of browns to choose from. You can mix shadow colors together for an optimum match. If you have black or brown hair you can brush it on with washable mascara.

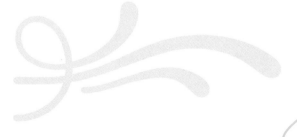

## The Wrong Color of Hair Dye

Tone down a too-bright color by massaging a few drops of olive oil into dry hair, then covering hair with a shower cap for thirty minutes. Shampoo with clarifying shampoo or even a mild dishwashing detergent.

## Emergency Hair Rescue for Long Hair

Part your hair down the center, and pull it back on either side. Make two tight braids from the ear to the nape of the neck, and secure them with rubber bands. Next, tease the ends with fingers, or use a brush to scrunch up ends so hair doesn't fall flat. Finish with your favorite hair spray.

## No Time to Dry

If you must run out of the house without blow-drying your hair, at least try to take a minute to dry from the top of your head to just above the ears. This is area that frames your face.

## Static Hair

If you ever find your hair catching on your coat or the walls, or that it stands on end when you attempt to brush it, always use a leave-in conditioner. If it's too late, slick on a bit of anti-frizz liquid.

For a last-minute fix, run a fabric softener sheet over your hair.

# Emergency Beauty Substitutions

Here are some products that can substitute for the original.

## No eye shadow

Substitute cream blush. Use your fingers to apply it. Stay with the bronze-toned blushes, not the red and pinks.

## Out of Eyeliner

Dip your eyeliner brush in waterproof mascara and apply.

## No Foundation

Take your concealer and mix it with moisturizer for a nice sheen.

## Emergency Blush

Use a pink-brown lipstick, dab on where needed, and blend with fingertips. Make sure the skin is moisturized.

## No Lipstick

Pour out some powder blush, then take a lip brush and mix it with a small dab of petroleum jelly. Apply with fingers.

## Unruly Eyebrows

Take a clean toothbrush or clean mascara wand, spray it with hairspray, and then brush the eyebrow up.

# Nail Emergencies

## Splitting Nail

Cut the nail, file it straight across, and then apply a couple of drops of nail glue to the surface of the nail. Let set and hold the break in place for about sixty seconds.

Reapply glue and then cover the nail with a piece of a tea bag or tissue.

Let dry, and then buff excess off.

## Emergency Nail Repair

When you've broken a nail and you really don't want to cut the other nails to match, purchase a set of preglued nails in a natural color. You can then set it on top of the broken nail and file and color to match your manicure.

## No Time for a Manicure

Rub olive oil on your nails when you don't have enough time to do a manicure.

The olive oil will give your nails smoothness and shine, and will soften torn and damaged cuticles.

## Caught Without a Nail File

Use a strip of a matchbook to file away snags.

# Clothing Emergencies

## Lint Remover

Use tape or a sticky label to remove lint. Use large mailer tape if you have it available.

## Stain Removal

Take a box of colored chalk and use it for these unforeseen emergencies.

When you have a stain, you can match the color of the stain with the color of the chalk.

Chalk washes out and won't ruin the fabric as some chemical removers can.

## Stuck Zipper

Use lip balm along the zipper teeth to unstick.

# chapter seventeen

# Common Beauty Questions

I get lots of mail, filled with lots of questions, and I pride myself on answering almost all of it. Here are some examples. Perhaps you have had one of these problems, and will be helped.

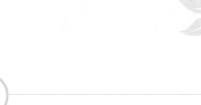

## [Q] *Dear Diane,*

How can I convince my wife that she is beautiful the way she looks? She is on the Internet every night and comes up with a new story of "how she should look."

Jim

## [A] **Dear Jim,**

I agree that beauty is not skin deep. It's attitude that separates the beauty from the crowd.

I have been privileged to work with models, actresses, and other celebrities who did not possess the physical characteristics of cookie-cutter beauty, but liked themselves so much that they lit a spark from within. Attitude is the first and most important issue and your wife needs to hear some positive enforcement. You're the perfect person to help. Don't go overboard, because it will sound insincere.

## [Q] Dear Diane,

I'm 29 and have developed dark shadow circles (not puffy) under my eyes. I have played around with concealers and yellow tinted concealers which are meant for dark circles but hate the "cakey" look. I feel that the concealers accent the fine lines. Is there a way to actually fade these circles? It seems that the circles are not surface skin level but under the skin.

*Kim*

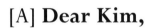

## [A] Dear Kim,

Apply vitamin K to this area. Gently "tap" it into the dark skin with your "pinky" finger.

I agree that the powder concealers look overly made up and accent every line. Here' a great trick. Take a small amount of yellow eye shadow and add it to your foundation. You'll disguise the darkness, and you can customize it to your skin type. If you don't want to use foundation, you can mix the yellow shadow with moisturizer.

## [Q] Dear Diane,

Are there any at-home remedies I can do to make my teeth whiter?

*Priscilla*

## [A] Dear Priscilla,

Mix baking soda and hydrogen peroxide and gently rub it into teeth, staying away from the gum area. Allow the solution to remain for about five minutes. Rinse. Don't use this treatment more than once a week.

## [Q ]Dear Diane,

My daughter recently joined a rugby team. Through the tackling, she has accumulated many bruises. Is there anything she can do to minimize the darkness of them, or to help speed up the healing process?

*Susan*

## [A] Dear Susan,

Horsetail extract, available at health food stores, can be applied to the bruise to help the healing. Look for it in capsule form. Prick one open with a pin, then spread the contents over the bruising.

## [Q] Dear Diane,

I am getting ready for my prom in a couple of weeks and I would love to do a really great makeup look on my eyes. Unfortunately my eyes always crease when I wear eye shadow. I've tried putting foundation on my eyes first, and certain base creams, but nothing works. I also want to use glitter.

*Joleen*

## [A] Dear Joleen,

Instead of foundation, apply dry face powder over the entire eyelid before applying shadow. Use a glitter stick and dot over the lid. Spread with your fingers. Line the upper and lower lids with pencil liner, and then seal it by going over it with a coordinating shadow.

## [Q] Dear Diane,

My fingernails are a reddish tint from wearing red nail polish. Is there anything I can put on them to make them a more natural color, or do I have to continue to cover them with colored polish?

*Wendy*

## [A] Dear Wendy,

Dissolve two denture cleanser tablets in a cup of warm tap water, and soak your hands in the mix. After a few minutes, wipe of the nail area with the combination of one teaspoon household bleach and one tablespoon warm water.

## [Q] Dear Diane,

What would you recommend to tighten up my loose neck? I wear turtlenecks so much I feel like a turtle. I don't want to resort to surgery. I'm 66 but I feel this neck makes me look much older.

*Jan*

## [A] Dear Jan,

Here's one of the facial exercises that I can recommend. Try to reach your nose with your tongue. Do this whenever you can, in the car, watching TV, or at your computer.

This silly-looking exercise will help tighten and build your neck muscles.

## [Q] Dear Diane,

I am starting to show signs of aging under my eyes. Is an eye moisturizer cream the only thing I should be using to help this?

*Penny*

## [A] Dear Penny,

The eyes are unfortunately the first to show signs of aging. If you don't want to pay for a pricey eye cream, then go to the drugstore and purchase vitamin A in oil or capsule form.

Find the highest concentration you can, and add it to your regular moisturizer. The ratio should be two-thirds vitamin A, one-third moisturizer. Gently "tap" the mixture into the area. Never rub cream around the eye area, where the skin is extremely delicate.

## [Q] **Dear Diane,**

I have a dandruff problem. I have already used several varieties of shampoos, but they don't seem to completely get rid of the dandruff. Can you help me solve this irritating problem?

*Lillith*

## [A] **Dear Lillith,**

Here's what models use to get rid of dandruff without altering their hair color. Take 30 uncoated aspirin and let them dissolve in a twelve-ounce bottle of basic drugstore shampoo. It is not necessary to refrigerate this bottle.

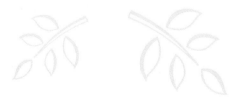

## [Q] **Dear Diane,**

Is there some trick with eye shadow I could do to minimize the appearance of my droopy eyelids? I'm 70 years old, which is what causes the problem. Even with droopy lids, my eyes are still my best feature and I would like for them to look their best.

*Joan*

## [A] **Dear Joan,**

I have a great secret for taking years off of your eyes. Apply neutral eye shadow or loose powder all over the eyelid. Then take a small eye shadow brush and draw a sideways "v" on the outer eye with a slightly darker shadow. Smudge it slightly. If you use eyeliner, powder over it with the same darker shadow.

Apply mascara at the roots, rather than the tip, to "open" the eye. Remember, practice makes you the expert. Always use a good magnifying mirror.

## [Q] Dear Diane,

I just learned that the school trip I will chaperone is scheduled as a sixteen-hour bus trip followed by an all-day visit to a theme park before we even see our hotel. Do you have any suggestions that will allow us to feel fresh?

*Joyce*

## [A] Dear Joyce,

Before you go, make up a strong cup of chamomile tea and place it in a small spritzer bottle. You can refresh both your face and reset your makeup throughout the trip. Also tuck a fabric softener sheet in your bag, and run it over your hair to tame the frizzies and keep your hairstyle in check. A couple of baby wipes will clean your skin and remove stains from your clothing.

## [Q] Dear Diane,

I am 39 and have a problem with the lines above my top lip. The wrinkles keep getting deeper. I keep looking older. Help me!

*Donna*

## [A] Dear Donna,

First, go to your local drugstore or health food store and purchase vitamin C powder.

Mix it with just enough moisturizer to make it spreadable, and then rub it into those lines with your finger. Follow up with the contents of a vitamin A capsule again tapped into this area and left overnight.

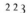

## [Q] Dear Diane,

I am 59 years young, and have fine hair. I have it foil-wrapped every two months. I feel I need a perm, but my hairdresser says NO. I have to curl my hair every day and it just doesn't hold a curl longer than a day. My hair is just to the end of my ears and is cut in layers. I tease it and tuck most of it behind my ears. I use a one-inch curling iron.

*Janet*

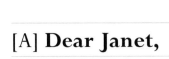

## [A] Dear Janet,

You can get a long-lasting curl without a curling iron and save your hair's health by taking a metal fork, twirling it around a strand of hair (just like spaghetti), and spritzing it with a bit of hair spray. Then you concentrate your hair dryer in that area and blow-dry the spray. The metal of the fork will seal your curl.

## [Q] Dear Diane,

I wonder if you can help me make a nose that is a little too wide (nostrils, that is) look thinner. I have a medium complexion and have tried a bit of eye shadow, but can't make it look natural.

*Betty*

## [A] Dear Betty,

No, eye shadow won't work, but a foundation or powder that is just one shade darker than your regular foundation will. Use it over the area that you wish to minimize and then take a separated tissue and blend over the area. Another option is to use bronzing powder. Again, don't choose a color that is more than two shades darker than your skin color.

## [Q] Dear Diane,

I am having a really hard time trying to get my hair to grow. Is there anything that can help?

*Joanne*

## [A] Dear Joanne,

Try adding flaxseed oil to your diet, which increases blood circulation to the scalp.

# eighteen

# Fabulous Figures

It doesn't matter what your body type, you owe it to yourself to feel comfortable in your skin. Whenever anyone comes to me with a desire to shape up their body, I insist that they work with me first to shape up their attitude. You need to appreciate the body you have to really know where you need to go to achieve your best form. Right now you need to start channeling your new body, and you need to do it without hiding out.

## No One Answer

Low-carb? Low-calorie? Combo eating? No matter what the plan, it will work for you if you have the right mindset. In all the years I've been in the beauty industry, I've found that there is no one plan that works for everyone. The best scenario is that you take the information from everything you've heard and work it into your own lifestyle. I don't know what you like to eat or what you're allergic to, and I've not interviewed any medical specialist who has convinced me that there is one answer.

## They're No Different

Celebrities and models gain and lose weight just like everyone else does. When they're not doing a movie or photo shoot they live real lives. So when you hear about them exercising five or six hours a day, it's because they are training for some event. What is different about these women that I've worked with is that they don't allow it to get out of hand. It's too hard to get back when they need to. The most successful bodies are the result of being in charge and knowing when to stop.

## Dieting Is Dead!

The idea is to change the way you look at food, so that you'll be healthier and stay thinner. Be intelligent about food, and be certain that whatever you eat you will end up wearing.

# What Do You Want to Weigh?

The weight ranges for men and women have recently changed. This is the latest chart to date. Realize that it's not just the pounds that count, it's how you carry them. If you are constantly trying to reach a goal that's five or ten pounds below what you currently weigh, then maybe you're not meant to be that weight. But first, look at your lifestyle. Is that Friday night pizza party more important than the fit of your jeans? It's a tough call that only you can answer.

| | |
|---|---|
| 5' 0" | 102–128 |
| 5' 1" | 106–132 |
| 5' 2" | 109–136 |
| 5' 3" | 113–141 |
| 5' 4" | 116–145 |
| 5' 5" | 120–150 |
| 5' 6" | 124–155 |
| 5' 7" | 127–159 |
| 5' 8" | 131–164 |
| 5' 9" | 135–169 |
| 5' 10" | 139–174 |
| 5' 11" | 143–179 |
| 6' 0" | 147–184 |

Heights are indicated for measurement without shoes.

Weigh yourself in the morning, before breakfast, and without any clothing.

## HEALTHY WEIGHT RANGES
## FOR MEN & WOMEN

# Top Secrets

## Ice Water

Ask any woman with a body to die for and most likely she will tell you that she drinks lots of water. That is so true, but it's only half the story. It's the ice that you add to your water that really makes the difference. Drinking ice water forces your system to rev up your metabolism to keep the body's temperature from dropping. For example, if you drink eight 12-ounce glasses of ice water a day, your body will burn an additional 200 calories. This does not apply to carbonated water.

Drink water consistently throughout the day. By the time you are really feeling thirsty, you are on your way to becoming dehydrated.

Often what we think of as hunger is thirst. If you find it difficult to down water in large quantities, flavor it up with a bit of lemon or lime. Water can provide a feeling of fullness, help the kidneys and liver do their job, and release toxins.

Don't be fooled into thinking that drinking lots of water will bloat you. Water retention is more likely to be caused by not drinking enough.

## Seeds

To maximize your intake of nutrients, add a lot of seed-containing fruits and vegetables such as apples, pears, and bananas, as well as the seeds themselves (like sesame or sunflower seeds). Seeds are a great source of fiber, allowing foods to go through your body quickly.

## Spicy Foods

Scientists have discovered that chili peppers, salsa, mustard, and ginger can actually raise your metabolic rate. The result is that you can burn calories much faster; up to 45 percent faster than that of a bland diet. How? These foods create a thermogenic burn, meaning they help the body to produce "heat," thus burning off calories.

## Herbs That Help Shed Pounds

There are herbs you can add to your diet as supplements, teas, and foods that will help your weight-loss program go smoothly. It's always smart to check with your doctor before adding any herb to your daily diet.

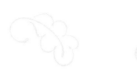
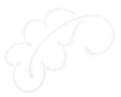

## Alfalfa

Aids digestion and acts as a diuretic.

## Bladder Wrack

Improves thyroid function and acts as a bulk laxative.

## Burdock

Improves fat metabolism and has diuretic effects.

## Cardamom

Improves circulation and digestion. A thermogenic herb.

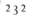

## Cayenne

Improves circulation and digestion. Has thermogenic effects.

## Cinnamon

Creates a thermogenic burn.

## Dandelion Root

Aids fat metabolism by affecting the liver.

## Fennel

A diuretic that reduces hunger and improves energy.

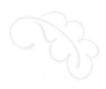

## Flaxseed

A bulk laxative that helps curb hunger.

## Garcinia Cambogia

Aids fat metabolism and reduces hunger.

## Green Tea

Aids fat metabolism and increases energy.

## Guar Gum

Helps to reduce hunger and has a laxative effect.

## Hawthorn

Reduces blood fat and improves circulation.

## Kola Nut

A stimulant that decreases appetite and aids in the metabolism of fat.

## Parsley

A diuretic and nutritional aid.

## Phyllium

Helps to curb hunger and allows the elimination of wastes from the body.

## Senna

An all natural laxative.

# Foods for the Skin

Think of food as a beauty aid. You want luxury!

## Blueberries

Promotes healthy collagen for fewer wrinkles. Less constriction of veins and faster healing.

## Carrots

Contains high levels of beta carotene for protection against sun damage.

## Salmon

Rich in essential fatty acids to keep skin moisturized.

## Eggs

High in the amino acid cystein, necessary for the growth and maintenance of the body's tissues.

## Yams

Rich in vitamin A to protect the skin from environmental damage.

## Mushrooms

Rich in selenium, an antioxidant that may help lower skin cancer risks.

## Yogurt

Contains vitamin B complex which is essential for smooth, blemish-free skin.

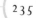

# Reasons to Eat Breakfast

You'll have a better day at work. Women who eat breakfast work faster and more accurately than those who don't. Breakfast eaters are also more creative in the morning.

It keeps you in shape. Breakfast eaters are slimmer than those who skip breakfast. They don't reach for doughnuts or croissants at the first coffee break.

You'll have lots of health benefits. Cereal with skim milk and fruit boosts your vitamin intake for under 200 calories.

# How to Get the Most from Your Meals

## Set a Beautiful Table

Choose one or two places in the home at which to eat. Make each meal a special occasion. Only eat at these places, and never eat while standing.

## Don't Play that Funky Music

Don't ever eat a meal to toe-tapping tunes. Researchers have found that diners who listen to classical music take three bites a minute versus five bites a minute for rock music. They also enjoy their meal more thoroughly and feel more satisfied.

## Just Eat

To be truly enjoyed, eating requires full attention. Turn off the TV, and put away that reading.

## Focus on Fragrance

Enjoy foods for their fragrance as well as their appearance and taste. Studies have proven that we obtain a great deal of satisfaction from a food's smell.

## Chew Away Tension

Relax your facial muscles and satisfy your chewing urges by chewing slowly. It takes fifteen minutes for your brain to communicate to your stomach that it's full.

## Small Is Smart

Choosing to eat meals on smaller, darker plates can fool the eye, which relates to tricking the brain into thinking that it's devoured a plateful.

## Add Flavor, Not Calories

Discover flavored vinegars to add flavor without the calories. Use a tablespoon of vinegar to thin down and extend your favorite dressings.

Add salsa to just about any food. It perks up the taste buds with little or no fat. Dip vegetables in it, spoon it over scrambled eggs, baked potatoes, and add it to salads.

Keep olive oil in a spritzer bottle and add it to salads, vegetables, and even popcorn.

## Say It with Soy

Soy is packed with powerful antioxidants that interfere with free-radical damage. This is the basis for how fast we age. Soy is another reason to turn to a more vegetarian-based diet. Unlike animal proteins, soybeans don't spew scads of damaging free radicals through your body to age your cells. Soy also prevents heart disease and diabetes. The Japanese, who eat the most soybeans in the world (thirty times more than Americans) live longer than anyone. Soy is also reported to cut breast cancer rates and to lower blood cholesterol.

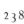

## Satisfy Your Sweet Tooth

When you desire something sweet, don't grab that candy bar. Try a natural sweet like grapes, blueberries, or strawberries.

When fruit just won't do, go for a jelly bean. At only six calories each, these fat-free sweets are one of the modeling world's favorite snacks. There are also sugar-free popsicles that have ten to fifteen calories that are a common snack for models.

## *How to Deal with Cravings*

## Brush Your Teeth

That awful taste you have in your mouth when restricting calorie intake can lead to eating. Instead, brush your teeth and tongue with a flavored toothpaste.

## Do Something Else

Take a bath or go to a movie. Take a walk or call a friend. Do anything until that hungry feeling goes away. Don't worry, eventually those cravings will subside.

## Drink Water

Add a lot of lemons to take away that awful empty feeling that cravings bring.

## Eat Bread

Sometimes a single slice of bread can calm nerves and end that craving like no other food can.

## Get Your Protein

A small protein-rich snack can eliminate that craving by keeping blood sugar and energy levels balanced.

## Rest

It may be that you just need to relax for a few minutes. Don't try to restore your energy level with food.

## Watch Out for Allergies

It may not be the food you're craving that's the culprit. Get checked for allergies to wheat and dairy.

# Are You Sure It's Hunger?

There are physical signs that will let you know if you're just experiencing a craving or if you're really hungry.

Headache, a lightheaded feeling, or irritability.

A need for any carbohydrate.

Increased salivation.

Stomach noises.

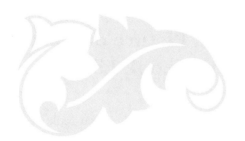

## Your Refrigerator

Did you know that the refrigerator is opened on an average of twenty-two times a day? Since it's such an integral part of our dining plans, here's how to make sure this appliance is not abused.

### Tack a Mirror on It

You can purchase a mirror that attaches to the front of the refrigerator. You'll find that if you have to face yourself each time you peek in, it just may wake you up to reality.

### Tape Up an Inspirational Note

Make that note a trigger for your success. "I can do it" or "Just a month until swimsuit season."

### Hang Up a Picture of What You Want to Look Like

It could be a photo of you when you looked your best. It might be a picture of your favorite celebrity.

Paste your head onto a supermodel's body.

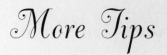

## Keep the Fat in the Fridge

Take one pound of butter or shortening and keep it in a plastic bag. Make it the first thing you see when you open that refrigerator.

## Portion All Your Foods

Pack all your food in bags. You'll see your daily allotment at a glance. Knowing that you're limited to those bags provides a focus.

## Red Wine

Drinking a glass of red wine can speed up metabolism rates.

## Lollipops

Sucking a lollipop can calm nerves and stop sugar cravings.

## Sugarless Candies

Candies and gums sweetened with artificial sweeteners can't be broken down in the body efficiently and can cause severe bloating.

## Stomachs Can Shrink

After a period of restricting calories, the stomach's capacity will actually decrease.

## Tensing

No need to stay at home with an expensive ab machine when you can tense your stomach muscles in and out wherever you are!

## The Fat Test

If you want to know if a food is high in fat but the container isn't around, rub the food with a paper napkin. If it leaves a grease mark, it probably has more fat than you want.

## Be Prepared

When traveling, always carry something healthy to eat and drink. It will steer you away from vending machines and fast-food restaurants.

# Cut Back on Calories without Counting

## Eat Treats

If you don't treat yourself now and then, you'll just crave it more. This will lead to an unfortunate binge.

## Leave Out the Fat

Chances are many of your favorite foods can remain in your diet if you cut back on cheese, butter, and cream.

## Spread It Out

Salad dressings and spreads can be thinned out with vinegars, yogurt, and other low-fat extenders.

## Check Your Portions

Weigh and measure your foods when it's convenient.

## Stop Late-Night Eating

Your body can't digest those late night snacks when it's at rest.

## Don't Drink Your Calories

Learn to like low-calorie drinks for painless calorie cutting.

## Don't Skip Meals

You'll end up eating twice as much, and your metabolism will be messed up with low blood-sugar levels.

## Shop with the Right Attitude

Never go shopping for food when you're ravenous. You'll end up with all the wrong stuff in your cart.

## What's In Your Coffee?

Since there are so many specialty coffees around, be certain that you're really ordering a potentially delicious, refreshing low-calorie drink.

| | |
|---|---|
| American drip | 4 calories |
| American decaf | 4 calories |
| Espresso | 5 calories |
| Cappuccino | 40 calories |
| Latte | 60 calories |
| Cafe mocha | 150 calories |

# Energize Your Fab Figure

## Cut Out Chemicals

Your body is not supposed to digest them. Processed food should always be the last option.

## Eat a Few Carbs

They feed the brain and can help you burn fat.

## Eat More Often

Even an ounce or two of protein like a slice of cheese or turkey can pick you up and keep your body from going into "starvation" state where it's trying to conserve every calorie.

## Condiments Count!

Ketchup and relish have unneeded calories. Mustard and lemon juice are better choices.

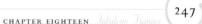

# *New Beauty*
# *Secrets*

# Face Treatments

## Lactic Acid Face Exfoliant

*It's not necessary to pay for expensive face exfoliants. Milk contains lactic acid, a gentle, yet effective, acid for getting rid of debris and damage to the top layer of the skin. The lemon juice allows the acid to penetrate the skin for maximum results.*

**1 tablespoon powdered milk**
**1 teaspoon lemon juice**
**1/2 teaspoon warm water**

1. Products should mix together to form a soft but spreadable paste.
2. Gently rub over the face working into the nasal and chin area.
3. Let set for a minute.
4. Rinse off with cool water.

## Oil-Absorbing Toner

*I use this toner before applying foundation to any client who has oily skin and needs to keep their makeup intact under hot lights (think runways, concerts) or for a special occasion (perfect for weddings).*

**1 teaspoon lemon juice**
**1 tablespoon witch hazel**
**1/4 teaspoon water**

1. Combine in a small bowl.
2. Swab all over face with a cotton ball or wash cloth, concentrating on the "T" zone.

# Cucumber Toner

*The cucumber contains refreshing and gently astringent properties. This makes it a wonderful treatment for the delicate skin around the eyes and the rest of the face.*

**1/2 small to medium cucumber cut into cubes (do not peel or seed)**
**2 tablespoons witch hazel**

1. Liquefy the cucumber in the food processor or blender.
2. Strain and mix cucumber juice with witch hazel.
3. Dip a cotton ball into the mixture and pat over eye area.
4. Take a small wash cloth and saturate with the remaining mixture.
5. Tap over entire face.

# Crow's Feet Treatment

*Vitamin A gently treats wrinkling around the eye while aloe vera allows for penetrating absorption.*

**1 vitamin A capsule**
**1 tablespoon aloe vera gel**

1. Blend the contents of the vitamin A capsule with the aloe vera gel.
2. Gently tap the mixture around the eye area with your pinky finger.
3. Apply at night and use with regular moisturizer.

## Face Puffiness Reducer

*Sometimes it's the way you slept, what you ate, or what you drank. On those mornings that you need to "depuff" your eyes or your entire face, rely on this behind the runway standby. The rose water tightens pores, while the chamomile tea reduces inflammation. The cold spoons calm down the puffiness.*

**1 cup chamomile tea, brewed with two tea bags**
**1/4 cup rose water**
**Small bowl filled with ice water**

1. Add the rose water to the cooled tea.
2. Dip cotton balls into mixture and dab generously over puffy areas.
3. Dip spoon into ice water and press metal over puffiness.

## Mashed Potato Neck Wrap

*This is a fantastic way of firming the neck area while using your leftovers!*

**1 cup mashed potatoes**
**Gauze padding**
**Hand towel**

1. If using cold mashed potatoes, briefly warm them in the microwave until just warm.
2. Spread over enough gauze to wrap completely around neck.
3. Gently place around neck and then cover over with warm towel.
4. Leave in place for about 20 minutes or until completely cool.
5. Rinse with warm water.
6. Follow with moisturizer.

## Basil Glow

*This is a wonderful herb for stimulating circulation and leaving skin absolutely glowing!*

**2 tablespoons of fresh basil**
   **or 1 teaspoon of dried basil**
**1 cup boiling water**

1. Brew the basil in the water until cool.
2. Pour into spritzer bottle and lightly spray over face.
3. Allow to air dry.

## Cuticle Softener

*This recipe will soften and condition the cuticle area. Resist the urge to use scissors.*

**2 tablespoons castor oil**
   **(available in drugstores)**
**2 tablespoons vegetable shortening**

1. Set both in the castor oil and vegetable shortening in a microwave-safe container.
2. Cook on high for 20 seconds.
3. Stir together and test to see that liquid is comfortable, yet warm to the touch.
4. Soak nails for 15 minutes.
5. Push back cuticles, then rinse.

## Make Your Own Body Powder

*This is a light, talc-free powder that feels wonderfully natural. Although this recipe traditionally uses almond extract, lemon or orange extract is just as good.*

**2 teaspoons cornstarch**
**3 tablespoons rice flour**
**5 to 6 drops pure almond extract**

1. Combine the cornstarch and flour.
2. Gradually add the almond extract.
3. Apply to body with a powder puff or large brush.

# Body

## Tension De-Stress Bath

*The warm scent of the almond oil relaxes the mind while the sesame oil and cinnamon soothe both skin and muscles.*

**1/2 cup sesame oil**
**1 tablespoon almond oil**
**1/2 teaspoon cinnamon**

1. Mix up ingredients with a fork and let stand for one hour.
2. Strain through paper towel.
3. Massage feet, hands, and any sore muscles.

## Acne Relief Body Treatment

**1 teaspoon geranium oil**
**1 teaspoon white iodine**
**1 teaspoon Epsom salts**

1. Mix all of the ingredients together in a small bowl.
2. With a cotton swab, apply to back acne, chest acne, and underarm acne.
3. Leave the mixture on for ten minutes, then wipe off with a warm, wet washcloth.

## Salt Scrub

*One of the most popular spa treatments is the salt scrub. It's a wonderful method of skin exfoliation and also stimulates body circulation to release toxins.*

**2 cups sea salt or kosher salt**
**1 cup olive oil**

1. Combine the salt and olive oil into a paste.
2. Rub on dry skin avoiding the neck and face.
3. Shower off.

## Home Spa Seaweed Wrap

*The number one spa treatment by far is the seaweed wrap. It sounds so exotic, and yet it is so easy to replicate in the privacy of your own bath.*

**1 package of dried seaweed (available in sheets at health food stores) or 1 cup powdered kelp**
**2 gallons water**
**1 beach towel**
**1 large plastic garbage bag, cut into a large rectangle**

1. Boil seaweed or kelp for five minutes.
2. Pour into large bowl.
3. Drop in towel and allow absorption of mixture.
4. Wrap towel around body and then wrap plastic bag over towel.
5. Rest for 15 to 20 minutes, then rinse.

# Beach Sand Elbow and Knee Exfoliant and Scrub

*Make a trip to the nearest beach and pick up a bucket of sand. Sand is a highly effective skin exfoliant, especially on resistant areas like knees and elbows.*

**2 tablespoons of beach sand or play sand**
**1 tablespoon of vegetable oil**
**1 sponge**

1. Boil the sponge in bleach and water to disinfect.
2. Take two tablespoons beach sand and mix with vegetable oil.
3. Massage on elbows and knees with hands or vegetable brush.
4. Rinse off with warm water and pat dry.

# Cuticle Softener

*Massage into cuticle area after manicure has fully dried. Not only will cuticles soften, but this solution will stimulate nail growth.*

**1 teaspoon olive oil**
**1 vitamin E capsule**

1. Combine ingredients in a small bowl.
2. Massage into nail bed and cuticles for five minutes, then rinse.

# Hair

## Moisturizing Jojoba Shampoo

*Jojoba oil has similar properties to our hair's natural oils. This enables it to help replenish the oils necessary for the health and shine of your hair.*

**1/2 cup water**
**1/3 cup regular shampoo**
**1 tablespoon Jojoba oil (available in drugstores and health food stores)**

1. Mix together in a bowl.
2. Use daily as a regular shampoo.

## Aspirin Scalp Treatment

*Use this mixture to get rid of dandruff and product buildup.*

**1 cup very hot water**
**30 uncoated aspirin tablets**
**1 tablespoon baking soda**

1. Dissolve aspirin in hot water.
2. Add baking soda and then allow to the mixture to cool until it's slightly warm.
3. Apply to clean wet hair, concentrating on scalp.
4. Leave on 20 minutes.
5. Rinse with warm water.

## Volumizing Shampoo

*Beer adds body and volume to hair and does not smell once it is rinsed out.*

**1 cup flat beer**
**1 teaspoon olive oil**

1. Mix beer and oil in a small bowl with a fork.
2. Pour mixture through hair and massage for two to three minutes.
3. Rinse and condition as usual.

## Paraffin Wax Treatment

*The most exclusive spas charge top dollar for this foot-softening paraffin wax treatment. Note: If you have trouble finding paraffin wax, you can substitute old candles.*

**4 bars of paraffin wax**
**1 bottle of rich moisturizer**

1. Melt the paraffin wax in a microwave.
2. Pre-moisturize feet and legs for protection.
3. Dip one foot into warm paraffin 3 times, pausing between layers to allow them to dry.
4. Wrap each foot with plastic wrap tight enough to make an airtight seal. This will help the moisturizer to penetrate.
5. Let set for 20 minutes.
6. Remove wrap and peel off the wax.
7. Rinse off with a coarse washcloth.

## *All-Day Lip Stain*

*This is used behind the runways and is the favorite way for models to keep their lips colored and flavorful!*

**1 envelope cherry or raspberry Jell-O**
**1 teaspoon petroleum jelly**

1. Melt petroleum jelly in microwave.
2. Mix in Jell-O.
3. Blend thoroughly and allow to cool.
4. Apply with a lipstick brush.

# Make Your Own Nail Polish

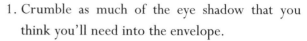

*This recipe is a great way to get just the color of nail polish you need, while getting rid of those extra-bold colored eye shadows you just don't dare to wear.*

**Eye shadow in your color choice**
**Paper envelope**
**Bottle of white nail polish**

1. Crumble as much of the eye shadow that you think you'll need into the envelope.
2. Snip off a corner of the envelope to make a tiny funnel.
3. Open the nail polish bottle and slowly pour the shadow into the polish.
4. Stir with the applicator until you get the desired color.
5. Make sure bottle is thoroughly mixed before applying.
6. You can touch up by mixing a very small amount of polish and shadow in a very small waxed paper cup.

# chapter twenty

# Final Thoughts

In the process of ending this book, I am considering what I hope you get from the many tips and ideas that you've just read. When I wrote the first *The World's Best-Kept Beauty Secrets*, it was my intention to reach the potential for everyone to discover not only their physical beauty, but the true beauty that lies within.

Today this is the thread, the intention, that runs through all my work. What you put in and on your body should make you feel as good as it makes you look. Otherwise it has no place in your life. That is really the biggest secret: that in beauty, diet, and especially style, anything that doesn't result in joy has no purpose.

Maintaining your best look should not be difficult and should not take too much time or money. It should never be a burden or responsibility to you or anyone in your life. It should bring you joy, lighten your heart, and allow you to feel better about yourself and the world around you. Most important, it should be fun.

You should approach beauty, diet, and fashion as self-care, a form of self-respect. You should care for yourself with the same reverence to the ones you love best. It's by doing that, by feeling and looking as good as you can that you can spread the joy and beauty to all that surrounds you.

What is the world's greatest beauty secret? In all my years of working in this industry I have decided that it's the appreciation of beauty in oneself and others that makes a woman truly beautiful. It is my final wish and heartfelt hope that you do the very best you can without obsessing, and that you spread beauty to others in all your words and acts.

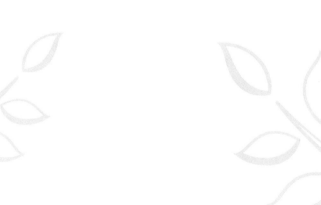

# Index

# About the Author

Diane Irons began her highly successful career as a model at age thirteen, then transferred her skills and expertise to training other up-and-coming models, as well as directing major photo shoots and runway shows. She continues to do so today while sharing her secrets with audiences throughout the world. As a leading force in the world of image, health, and fitness, she is frequently featured on *The View, Good Morning America, Entertainment Tonight, Inside Edition,* and CNN, and in publications worldwide.

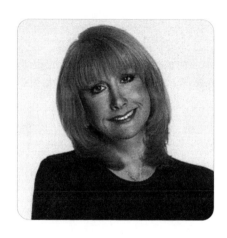

For more information, please see Diane's website at www.DianeIrons.com

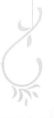